The Sa

Cook Book

Emil G. Conason and Ella Metz

ISBN: 1530077737
ISBN-13: 978-1530077731

CONTENTS

INTRODUCTION

THE body fluids of man contain precisely 0.85% of salt.
This percentage of salt is maintained in the blood of all healthy
individuals. Any radical change in its proportion will cause catastrophic,
life-threatening changes in the blood elements. A marked increase in
concentration in the blood causes the red blood cells to shrink and
wrinkle. A lowering of the normal percentage causes swelling and then
rupture of the red blood cells.
Common table salt, chemically, is sodium chloride. A molecule of salt is
made up of an atom of sodium joined to an atom of chlorine. This
chemical combination formed by the union of the soft, lustrous, silver-
like metal, sodium, and the greenish yellow, acrid, poisonous gas,
chlorine, has always been considered one of the most innocuous of all
the substances consumed by living matter. Practically all living matter
contains salt. Without it life would seem to be impossible. In many parts
of the world there are great salt licks to which the local wild
life periodically is attracted to replenish its salt needs. Some powerful
instinct seems to lead animals to the salt supply. Among some of the
pygmy tribes of Africa whose normal terrain is lacking in salt, the
mineral has become a prized symbol of wealth and a means of exchange.
The exchange of foods and waste materials by the living cells of the
body depends upon the concentration of sodium on the cell membrane.
Any shift of serious proportions in the body's salt concentration causes
interference with normal metabolism of the cells and eventually causes
death of the tissues themselves. Research has shown that it is the sodium
ion and not the chloride ion which is responsible for water retention in
the body. The mechanism by which the concentration of salt is kept at
the physiological point is by way of the kidneys. If salt tends to increase
in concentration in the blood, urination increases and the excess salt is
excreted through the urine. Any tendency to dropping of the salt level of
the blood is, offset by kidney retention. The ability of the kidney to
keep, the salt concentration in balance depends in its turn on
the functioning of the adrenal cortex gland. This eland
excretes hormones into the blood which tend (among other things) to
keep the ratio of sodium, potassium and calcium at the proper level. In
disease involving the adrenal cortex, the heart, the liver, or the kidney
itself, the normal balance of the body sodium is violently changed. With

4

the change in sodium balance, a resulting change in water balance also occurs. The tissue spaces become water-logged or edematous. Fluids gather in unaccustomed places; organs are swollen out of all proportion; their functions interfered with; and a vicious cycle of degeneration is set up. The swollen kidney or liver or brain fails to function properly. The edematous adrenal cortex is less able to bring about the normal kidney exchange; the heart finds difficulty in pumping the blood through the waterlogged tissue spaces; cellular respiration is interfered with; tissues die. Whichever organ system is initially at fault, all organs and all body tissues are finally involved unless some way is found to restore the balance and clear the body of the retained sodium and its attendant water. The healthy individual, averaging 150 lbs., normally excretes 10 to 15 grams (10,000-15,000 milligrams) of sodium chloride every 24 hours (since sodium constitutes roughly 51% of sodium chloride, that is, 5 to 8 grams of sodium per day). It is obvious that to do this he must consume in his food and drink a similar quantity of sodium chloride. As I have remarked above, in the healthy individual any sudden increase in the daily sodium intake results in an increased output of salt by way of the urine; likewise, a marked diminution in the intake of sodium results in retention by the kidneys and a decrease in urination. Not so in those whose physiological mechanisms are unbalanced. In the sick, salt often tends to accumulate and to hold water in the tissue spaces. From the point of advantage of the backward glance one is tempted to express amazement at the failure of medical science to recognize earlier the importance of regulating sodium intake in the control of such conditions as:

1. Dropsy (the edema of cardiac failure)
2. Nephritis
3. Nephrosis
4. The edema of liver cirrhosis
5. Meniere's syndrome (ringing in the ears and dizziness)
6. Eclampsia (the toxemia of pregnancy)
7. In pre-menstrual tension
8. Migraine
9. Epilepsy
10. In intractable insomnia and nervous tension states
11. Rheumatic arthritic swelling
12. Hypertension (high blood pressure)
13. Reducing diets

However, it was not until the early 1920's that attention was called to the possibility of breaking the vicious cycle of sodium and water retention and imbalance. In the same year (1922) that saw the mass commercial production of insulin for diabetics, Dr. Frederick M. Allen and his co-workers announced the use of a diet low in sodium chloride as a treatment for hypertension (high blood pressure). This group treated 280 patients suffering with very severe, otherwise uncontrollable, high blood pressure with a diet in which the sodium content was held down to 150 milligrams. They followed their cases for a period of over 4 years. They were convinced that those who adhered to the diet were vastly improved in health and that their lives had been greatly prolonged. Allen's follow-up of the low-sodium diet treatment of severe hypertensives in the past quarter century has so completely convinced him of the value of the treatment that he recently summed up his experiences in a discussion reported in the Journal of the American Medical Association, June 4, 1949, page 462. Recognizing the fact that there were a few patients who were refractory to treatment, Allen goes on to say: "Just as in diabetes, failure in worst cases do not invalidate diet principle. My distinction 22 years ago between symptom and disease of hypertension, explains benefits, not merely measured by pressure reduction and often apparent after years in initially refractory cases.... Diet keeps all but extremely hypertensive patients active and improved. Frequent clearing of retinitis (swelling of the retina and optic nerve of the eye), congestive failure (heart failure), headache, dyspnea (shortness of breath) and other symptoms is unmistakable.... Appetizing diet encourages fidelity. Long ago, the public should have been taught to accept diet for hypertension as routinely as for diabetes. The waste of life during the past twenty years may continue for another 10 years before all agree. My conclusion, based on unique experience in several thousand cases during twenty-eight years, is that saltless diet, especially when begun reasonably early can specifically arrest progressiveness, prevent complications, and thus provide the first real control of deaths from hypertension."

During the past few years there has been a new flurry of attention to the use of the low sodium diet in high blood pressure. Dr. Walter Kempner, assistant professor of clinical medicine at Duke University, Durham, N. C., has enthusiastically reported great success in the treatment of patients with high blood pressure by the so-called Rice Diet. In this diet, as in Dr. Allen's diet, the sodium content is held down to 150 milligrams. At a meeting of the New York Heart Association, Nov. 16, 1948, Dr. Kempner reported the results in his treatment of 700 patients. His Rice Diet was given to these patients for periods ranging between 35 and 900 days. He reports beneficial effects in 70 percent of his patients.

THE RICE DIET

Dr. Kempner's diet is called the Rice Diet because it is based upon rice as one of its main constituents. The diet contains in some 2000 calories only 20 grams of protein and 5 grams of fat per day. As mentioned above no more than 150 milligrams of sodium is permitted in the 24 hours. The rice, which forms the backbone of the diet, may be brown, polished or wild. Fruit is used to supplement the rice. So long as it is unsalted, the fruit may be raw, stewed, canned, dried, frozen or preserved. Nuts, dates and avocados are forbidden. While brown or white sugar or honey may be used none of the ordinary commercial syrups, such as Karo or maple syrup are permitted. Vegetable juices are NOT included. Fluids are limited to a pint and a half to two pints of fruit juices (canned or fresh). The following supplement completes the diet:

Vitamin A	5000	units
Vitamin D	1000	units
Riboflavin	5	milligrams
Thiamin Chloride.	5	milligrams
Niacinamide	25	milligrams
Ferrous Sulphate	0.6	milligram

Dr. Kempner is careful to state that while the usual caloric intake of the patients is restricted to 2000 calories, he often finds it necessary to vary the calories according to the patient's need to gain or lose weight. He points out that the average time required for attaining a marked decrease in blood pressure is between 3 and 4 months. He has seen marked decreases in as little as 4 days. An occasional patient has taken 12 months. Dr. Kempner claims that the Rice Diet, under his supervision, has resulted in significant reduction in the size of greatly enlarged hearts and that the edema (water logging of the tissues) due to kidney disease was eliminated. He has also commented on favorable changes in electrocardiograms and favorable changes in the fundus of the eye (retina and optic nerve head). In Dr. Kempner's papers the striking effects of the Rice Diet on heart size, blood pressure, electrocardiographic markings and on the ocular fundi have been seen most often in patients with congestive heart failure or nephritis.
OTHER LOW SODIUM DIETS The diets of both Allen and Kempner are so rigid that they Association June 4, 1949, page 462) undertook to

study a group of patients who were ambulatory. They put these patients on are not feasible in the ambulatory patient. Dr. Milton Landowne and his co-workers (Journal of the American Medical a diet limited to 300 milligrams of sodium per day. Unknown to the patient he was given 2 grams (2000 milligrams) of sodium a day in a capsule. Urinary studies of sodium output showed that only one in three patients stayed within the lim its of the diet despite the fact that their actual daily sodium intake was far beyond that permitted in the rice diet or in Allen's diet. Their sodium intake was more than 2300 milligrams per day. It would seem obvious that such results as Allen and Kempner achieved can be reproduced only under the rigid supervision made possible by hospital care.

Nevertheless a number of reports have been made on the advantages and beneficial effects of other low sodium diets in various conditions. For instance, M. H. Barker reports on the beneficial effects in patients with congestive heart failure of a diet containing 1000 milligrams of sodium a day. (Journal of the American Medical Association, June 1932). F. R. Schemm in the Annals of Internal Medicine, Dec. 1942, reports benefit in cardiac edema patients with a diet containing somewhat over 1,000 milligrams of sodium per day.

The famous Karrell Diet which consisted of 4 glasses of milk with 8 slices of dry salt-free toasted bread per day, was used in cardiac and nephritic edema with great success by the doctors of the early 20tn century. Its benefits might well have been due to the fact that the total sodium intake of such a diet is about 600 milligrams.

Wheeler, Bridges and White (Journal of the American Medical Association Jan. 4, 1947, pages 16-20) treated congestive heart failure in a series of 50 patients with a diet containing about 625 milligrams of sodium. Their patients were selected because of their refractoriness to previous therapy. Of the 50 patients, 35 had faithfully followed the diet. Of these 22 were improved, 13 showed no improvement. Walsh and Adson (Journal of the American Medical Association Jan. 13, 1940, pages 130-136) treated 128 patients suffering with Meniere's syndrome on low sodium diet. They gave their patients ammonium chloride to increase urinary output. Forty-five of these patients were completely relieved of their vertigo. Thirty-three reported vertigo improved. Fifty patients found no improvement. M. M. Miller (Journal of the American Medical Association Sept. 22, 1945, pages 262-266) treated 20 patients suffering from insomnia ana nervous tension. He used a diet restricted to 2 grams (2000 milligrams) of sodium chloride a day. Seventeen of these patients reported that their symptoms disappeared under treatment. When 13 of these patients were placed on a normal salt intake, relapses occurred in 10 of them. K. De Snoo, in the American Journal of Obstetrics and Gynecology Dec. 1937, implicated sodium as the cause of the eclampsia of pregnancy. He advocated a low-salt diet in pregnant women during the second half of pregnancy. J. O. Arnold in the Medical Clinics of North America July 1934, had suggested the limitation of salt in the diet of pregnant women threatened with eclampsia.

W. Pomerance and I. Daichman, American Journal of Obstetrics and Gynecology Dec. 1940, make the interesting ob servation that the length of labor is apparently reduced by a low salt diet in the latter part of pregnancy. Greenhill and Fried, Journal of the American Medical Association Aug. 16, 1941, and Thom et al, Endocrinology Feb. 1938, found benefit in low-sodium diets in the edema and tension of the so-called premenstrual state.

HOW THESE MENUS SHOULD BE USED

It is of course assumed that patients who are in need of the low-sodium menus outlined in this book are under the care of a competent doctor. The patient is strongly urged to check frequently with his doctor. The constant check-up is just as important in the low-sodium diet as it is in diabetes. In such conditions as Addison's disease, a disease of the adrenal cortex, sodium deprivation may actually initiate collapse. Occasional urine analysis for sodium or chloride content will guide the doctor in his prescription of the various sodium levels. For instance, in the case of the cardiac patient whose water retention has been relieved by rigid adherence to the Rice Diet, the doctor may find it desirable to raise the sodium content to a 300 milligram level per day for maintenance; likewise in patients with nephrosis, Meniere's syndrome, and even hypertension. Surely the pregnant patient who has been delivered of her child will want her sodium intake allowance raised to the highest point consistent with good health. The division of our suggested menus at varying sodium levels is meant to be of assistance to the doctor in his prescribing. We suggest that the doctor use his judgment in varying the menus, eliminating where he finds it desirable, combining elements from each group and improvising where he finds it possible to take the time. To take but a simple example, the elimination in our Menu 1 for breakfast of ½ cup of milk, reduces the sodium content of the breakfast from 81.4 to 23.4 milligrams of sodium.

We have attempted to make this book a manual of convenience for both the doctor and the patient. Our special menus for the diabetic who

9

requires low-sodium intake, for the person who eats out, for the obese patient who requires weight reduction, are each subject to interchange and modification. For the doctor who wishes to make his own changes we have added a table at the end of the book of the sodium content of hundreds of the commonly used basic foods. It will be noted that four authorities, whose findings are extremely divergent as to sodium content of the same foods, are quoted. This has not been done with the intent to confuse the reader. The confusion among scientists and in the scientific literature, and the difference in chemical estimation, have been due to the fact that until very recently there were no accurate tests available for the estimation of sodium as such. The various scientific writers on diet and nutrition were forced to make highly inaccurate indirect estimates of sodium content This was usually done by careful chemical estimations of the chlorides present. From the chloride content the sodium content was then assumed. We have found the book, The Chemical Composition of Foods by R. A. McCance and E. M. Widdowson published by the Chemical Publishing Co., Inc., Brooklyn, N. Y., fairly consistent and in general agreement with the figures quoted in the special brochure published by Mead Johnson & Co., Evansville 21, Indiana entitled Sodium and Potassium Analysis of Foods and Waters. The figures quoted by Mead Johnson were obtained by the special process of flame photometry. The analysis was made by their own research laboratories. Wherever we have used a figure in which there was disagreement between these two authorities, we have taken the higher figure on the assumption that it was desirable to err if necessary on the side of a lower rather than a higher sodium content. Where either of these two authorities failed to give the figure for sodium in a food, we have resorted to Chemistry of Food and Nutrition, by Henry C. Sherman, Ph.D., Sc.D., published by the Macmillan Co., New York, and on Elements of Food Biochemistry by Peterson, Skinner and Strong, published by Prentice-Hall, Inc., New York.

Throughout the book we have placed side by side the caloric value and the sodium value in milligrams per ounce of the various foods and combinations we have used. We have expressed these measurements in milligrams per ounce and in calories per ounce. For the benefit of those who prefer to use the metric system throughout rather than the hybrid method we have chosen, milligrams per ounce as well as calories per ounce may be roughly translated to milligrams and calories per hundred grams by merely multiplying each of our figures by 30.

All recipes are given in single portion quantities unless otherwise stated. Wherever, in the menus, recipes are given for certain dishes, the fact is denoted by the presence of an asterisk after the name of the dish.

The preparation of palatable menus for the patient requiring sodium restriction was far from simple. In attempting to treat a number of patients who found it impossible to adhere to the stringent rigidities of the Rice Diet, I discovered the lack of any available source of information for the patient's use. As patient after patient complained of the colorlessness and inanity of the diets I prescribed, and as their urine chloride tests showed more and more frequent lapses in their adherence to the diet, the need for this book became apparent
My colleague, Miss Ella Metz, undertook to work out a practical, kitchen-wise, helpful, series of more interesting menus to meet this need. Each of the dishes has been actually prepared and served to a member of her family in need of low-sodium diet This book is the result.
Emil G. Conason, M.D.

Table of Measurements

All measurements are given as level measurements

3 teaspoons	1	tablespoon
4 tablespoons	¼	cup
8 tablespoons	½	cup
16 tablespoons	1	cup
1 cup	1	glass
2 cups	1	pint
4 cups	1	quart
4 quarts	1	gallon

Table of Weights

1 cup, liquid	8 oz.
2 cups, liquid	1 lb.
2 cups sugar	1 lb.
½ cup butter or 8 T. butter	¼ lb.
4 cups flour	1 lb.
1⁷⁄₈ cups rice	1 lb
No. 1 can	1¹⁄₃ c.
No. 2 can	2½ c.

No. 2½ can	3½ c.
No. 3 can	4 c.

Table of Abbreviations

ave	average	Na	sodium
btl	bottle	OZ	ounce
bx	box	Prot	proteins
cal	calories	pkg	package
Carb	carbohydrates	pt	pint
ch	chop	sl	
diam.		sm	
hd	head	st	
lb		str	
larg	large	T	tablespoon
mg		t	

A Basic Group of Low Sodium Foods

Beverages
Coca Cola, Cocoa, Coffee, Fruit Juices, Tea, Ginger Ale, Wines, Postum
Condiments
Allspice, Caraway, Cinnamon, Curry powder, Garlic, Mace, Mustard
powder, Nutmeg, Paprika, Pepper, Peppermint extract, Sage,
Thyme, Tumeric, Vanilla extract, Vinegar,

Avoid onion salt, celery salt and garlic salt. Also avoid all prepared
flavorings like prepared horse radish, prepared mustard, Worcestershire
Sauce, etc.

Fats and Oils
Beef dripping, Butter unsalted, Crisco, Olive oil, Salad oil
Avoid margarine, salted butter, bacon fat, and other fats to which salt has
been added.

Cereals and Cereal Foods

Arrowroot, Barley pearl, Cornflour, Cracked
Wheat, Cornmeal, Farina, Flour—white, Flour—Wheatmeal, Macaroni,
Maltex, Oatmeal, Puffed Rice, Puffed Wheat, Rice, Sago, Semolina,
Shredded Wheat, Soya flour, Tapioca, Wheatena

Dairy Products — Most dairy products are high in sodium. The
following are lower than most:.

	mg. per oz
Butter	1.4
Cream	11.4
Egg yolk..............	14.2
Milk.....................	14.5

Meat Products—Most meat products are high. The following are the
ones containing the least amount of sodium.

	mg. per oz.		mg. per oz.
Beef, lean	19.6	Rabbit, foreleg	13.4
Chicken, breast	22.2	Rabbit, loin	9.7
Durk. breast	19.4	Sweetbreads	19 6
Hare.	15.0	Tripe	13.1
Lamb, lean	31.4	Turkey breast .	11.4
Liver, beef	24.4	Turkey, leg.	26.2
Pig pancreas	16.2	Veal	30.4
Pigeon	21.0	Venison	24.4
Pork, lean	18.8		

Note: Avoid all smoked and processed meats. Frozen meats may be used
if not salted.

Fish
All fish except shellfish, may be used, with the exception of oysters.
Avoid all salted and smoked fish.

Fruits
All fruits and juices, canned or fresh. Avoid those that have sodium
benzoate or salt added.

Nuts
All nuts except those that are salted.

Vegetables
Most fresh and canned, except those that have sodium benzoate or salt added (see listing of canned vegetables prepared without salt at end of this section. Avoid celery, beets, dandelion, kale, mustard greens, spinach and sauerkraut.

Sugar and Preserves
Chocolate Plain, Coconut dry, Sugar, Honey, Jam, Jelly, Marmelade

INTRODUCTION TO LOW SODIUM MENUS

General Rules to Follow in Using Recipes

No salt is to be added to any recipe.
All butter used is to be entirely salt free.
No margarine is to be used for shortening. Use only vegetable oils, butter, unsalted, or beef drippings, unsalted.
Canned fruits may be used if no sodium benzoate has been added.
Since canned vegetables are often packed with salt, none are to be used except where noted.
In some cities low sodium bread may be purchased in chain bakeries. This bread or matzoths may be substituted for the bread recipes on the menus.
Quantities given are for one serving only, unless otherwise stated. Many readers will wish to increase the amounts to save waste, as for example, when ½ egg is required the recipe can be double and two portions made.
In boiling, many foods lose some of their sodium. However, this loss is sustained only if the liquor in which the food was boiled is not used.
The drinking of water should be controlled if local water supply is high in sodium. In such instances distilled water may be used.

MENUS 1-10

400 - 500 Milligrams of Sodium 1800 - 2200 Calories
Measurements are expressed in milligrams of sodium and
calories in each portion

MENU 1
Breakfast

	Milligrams Sodium	Calories
8 oz. Orange Juice (1 cup)	4.0	88
¼ cup Oatmeal (1 oz.) with	9.5	115
½ cup milk	58.0	76
1 cup Coffee, with		8
2 t. cream	3.8	38
1 t. sugar		19
1 sl. Low Sodium Bread*	3.5	97
½ T. Marmalade or Jelly	2.6	37
	81.4	478

Lunch

	Milligrams Sodium	Calories
Scrambled Eggs and Mushrooms*	81.1	130
Salad — ½ banana, ½ apple sliced, 1 large lettuce leaf shredded.	5.1	56
Orange Rice Custard*	30.6	409
	116.8	595

(When making Custard, boil one T. rice for breakfast tomorrow)

Dinner

	Milligrams Sodium	Calories
½ lb. Broiled Beef Liver	195.2	328
1 Baked Potato, medium	8.0	96
1 t. butter (unsalted)	0.2	38

15

4 oz. String Beans, Creole*	15.0	114
Salad—2 oz. lettuce and I medium tomato	10.0	22
Vinegar Dressing*	3.0	63
Baked Apple with	2.4	40
1 t. sugar and cinnamon		19
Coffee—1 t. sugar and 2 t. cream	3.8	65
	237.6	785
Total for Day	435.8	1858

*Asterisks denote dishes for which recipes are given.

RECIPES FOR MENU 1

LOW SODIUM BREAD

	Milligrams Sodium	Calories
½ cake yeast (½oz.)	0.5	13
½ T. sugar		28
½ cup milk	58.5	76
1 T. Spry (or other vegetable shortening)		110
3½ cups flour (about)	9.6	1600
1 T. melted butter	0.7	113
½ cup water		
	69.3	1940

Crumble the yeast, and add sugar. Heat the water, milk and shortening together in a saucepan. Add this to the yeast and sugar and mix well. Add half the flour and mix well. Add the remainder of the flour to make a stiff dough. Knead the dough until smooth and place in greased bowl. Spread melted shortening over dough. Cover with towel and let rise in warm place until double in size. Knead again and shape into loaves. Place in well greased loaf pan and spread with melted shortening. Cover and let rise again until double in bulk. Bake in a moderately hot oven for 1 hour. This loaf will yield about 20 slices of bread. One slice equals 3.5 mg. sodium and 97 calories.

SCRAMBLED EGGS AND MUSHROOMS

	Milligrams Sodium	Calories
½ cup mushrooms (about 1²/₃ oz.)	4.3	3
1 t. butter	0.2	38
1 egg 67.0		77
4 t. milk	9.6	12
pepper		
	81.1	130

Sauté mushrooms in butter for a few minutes. Place in top of double boiler. Add egg, milk, and pepper. Cook slowly, stirring until creamy.

ORANGE RICE CUSTARD

	Milligrams Sodium	Calories
1 T. rice	1.2	68
3 T. light cream	17.1	172
2 t. sugar		38
4 t. orange juice	0.3	8
2 T. heavy cream	11.4	115
4 t. water and bit of orange rind		
¼ orange in sections	0.6	8
	30.6	409

Place washed rice, water and light cream in top of double boiler. Cover and steam until rice is tender. Add sugar, orange juice and rind. Cool. Whip cream (heavy) and fold into the mixture. Pour into cups and chill. Unmold and trim with orange sections.

STRING BEANS CREOLE

	Milligrams Sodium	Calories
¾ cup string beans (4 oz.)	7.2	16
1 small onion—2 oz	5.8	14
½ tomato	1.6	8
2 t. shortening (butter)	0.4	76

15.0   114

Cut one small onion and brown lightly with the shortening. Slice in ½ tomato. Put in string beans and a little water. Cook on small flame until tender (about 20 min.).

VINEGAR DRESSING

	Milligrams Sodium	Calories
1 T. vinegar	3.0	
1 t. olive oil		44
1 t. sugar		19
	3.0	63

MENU 2
BREAKFAST

	Milligrams Sodium	Calories
4 oz. Orange Juice (½ cup) with ½ Banana, sliced	2.5	77
1 T. Rice (cooked the night before when making Orange Rice Custard)	1.2	68
½ cup Milk, hot, with rice	58.0	76
1 t. Sugar and Cinnamon may be added to Milk		19
1 slice Low Sodium Bread (see Menu 1)	3.5	97
2 t. Jelly	4.8	49
	73.8	451

LUNCH

	Milligrams Sodium	Calories
1 Fried Egg and Mashed Potato	72.8	249
4 oz. Boiled Fresh Asparagus	2.0	20
1 T. Melted Butter (unsalted)	0.6	114

	3.5	97
1 slice Low Sodium Toast (see Menu 1)	3.5	97
1 cup Fruit Salad (canned) 4 oz	10.0	80
Coffee—2 t. cream, 1 t. sugar	3.8	65
	92.7	625

DINNER

	Milligrams Sodium	Calories
½ Grapefruit	0.8	12
½ lb. Broiled Shoulder Lamb Chops, lean only (weighed with fat and bone)	136.0	288
4 oz. Fresh Peas, boiled		56
1 Boiled Parsley Potato	4.0	92
Salad, 1 oz. cucumber, ½ tomato, 1 oz. lettuce	8.7	14
4 t. Vinegar Dressing (see recipe Menu I)	3.0	63
Cocoanut Cream Tapioca*	88.4	326
Coffee—2 t. cream, 1 t. sugar	3.8	65
	244.7	916
Total for Day	411.2	1992

RECIPES FOR MENU 2

FRIED EGGS AND MASHED POTATOES

	Milligrams Sodium	Calories
1 potato, boiled and mashed	4.0	92
1 T. onion shredded	1.4	92
1 egg	67.0	77
2 t. butter	0.4	76
	72.8	249

Fry onions in butter. When onions are browned, remove them and fry eggs in onion flavored butter. Boil and mash the potato. Garnish the potato with the browned onions and serve with the egg.

COCOANUT CREAM TAPIOCA (It is best to make this recipe for four portions)

	Milligrams Sodium	Calories
2 t. tapioca (⅓ oz.)	0.4	34
1 T. sugar	0.5	56
¼ egg	17.0	19
1 T. shredded coconut	1.1	26
½ cup milk	58.0	76
2 T. cream	11.4	115
Few drops vanilla		
	88.4	326

MENU 3

BREAKFAST

	Milligrams Sodium	Calories
Mix 4 oz. orange and 4 oz. of grapefruit juice	2.8	56
1 Shredded Wheat biscuit (1 oz.) with	4.7	103
½ Banana (2½ oz.) with	0.5	33
½ cup milk	58.0	76
1 slice Toasted Low Sodium Bread (see Menu 1) with	3.5	97
1 t. butter (unsalted)	0.2	38
Coffee—2 t. cream, 1 t. sugar	3.8	65
	73.5	468

LUNCH

	Milligrams Sodium	Calories
Spanish Omelet*	93.0	136
1 slice Low Sodium Bread	3.5	97
1 t. butter (unsalted)	0.2	38
Nut and Apple Tapioca*	8.5	409
Coffee with 1 t. sugar and 2 t. cream	3.8	65

	109.0	745

DINNER

	Milligrams Sodium	Calories
Salmon Steak*	242.6	487
Baked Potato with 1 t. Butter	8.2	134
Diced Carrots with Minted Peas*	28.9	65
Hearts of Lettuce (2 oz.)	6.8	6
1 T. French Dressing*		88
Pineapple and Cocoanut*	3.4	123
	289.9	903
Total for Day	472.4	2116

RECIPES FOR MENU 3
SPANISH OMELET

	Milligrams Sodium	Calories
1 egg	67.0	77
½ onion (1 oz.)	2.9	7
1 oz. green pepper (3" piece)	0.1	8
½ cup tomatoes (unsalted, 4 oz. canned)	20.4	24
2 fresh mushrooms, peeled and washed (1 oz.)	2.6	2
Few fresh green peas		18
	93.0	136

Cut up onion, green pepper. Add tomatoes, green peas and
cut-up mushrooms. Cook until soft. Season before serving with a
little pepper. Make plain omelet and put in filling when finished.

NUT AND APPLE TAPIOCA

	Milligrams Sodium	Calories
2 T. pearl tapioca	0.9	68
½ cup water		
1 T. sugar	0.5	9
2 T. chopped walnuts	0.8	208

	Milligrams Sodium	Calories
1 T. cream	5.7	58
½ t. sugar		9
2 T. apples diced (1 oz.)	0.6	10
Bit of vanilla		
	8.5	409

Soak tapioca in water for several hours. Add sugar and apples and cook until tapioca is tender and mixture is thick, about 1 hour. Add nuts, cool and serve with sweetened flavored cream.

SALMON STEAK

	Milligrams Sodium	Calories
2 small mushrooms, chopped fine	2.6	2
½ oz. minced onion	0.9	2
1 t. minced parsley		
2 t. butter	0.4	76
1/3 wine glass sherry (1 oz.)	2.8	24
1 T. fine bread crumbs (1/3 oz)	38.3	15
½ lb. fresh salmon (weighed with bones)	197.6	368
	242.6	487

Sprinkle salmon with mushrooms, onion and parsley. Dot with butter. Add sherry and bake in moderate oven, in shallow baking dish, for 15 min. Then sprinkle with the crumbs and continue baking another 15 min. basting several times.

DICED CARROTS WITH MINTED PEAS

	Milligrams Sodium	Calories
1 diced carrot (2 oz.)	28.4	10
1/3 cup green peas (2 oz.)	0.5	36
½ t. butter		19
Bit of mint, crushed		
	28.9	65

Cook diced carrots until tender. Cook peas with crushed mint. When ready to serve combine carrots and peas and melted butter.

FRENCH DRESSING (makes ¾ cup)

	Milligrams Sodium	Calories
½ garlic clove		
½ cup olive oil		1056
Few grains paprika, few grains pepper		
3 T. lemon juice	0.6	3
	0.6	1059

1 T. equals 88 calories

Make cuts in clove of garlic. Rub bowl with it and then leave it in bowl. Add other ingredients. Stir vigorously with fork. Let stand 30 min. Remove garlic. Beat dressing thoroughly. Keep in refrigerator.

PINEAPPLE AND COCOANUT

	Milligrams Sodium	Calories
4 oz. canned pineapple chunks	1.1	72
2 T. moist coconut (1/7 oz.)	2.3	51
	3.4	123

Mix ingredients thoroughly and serve chilled.

MENU 4
BREAKFAST

	Milligrams Sodium	Calories
8 oz. Orange Juice	4.0	88
1 cup Puffed Rice (½ oz.)	0.1	60
½ cup Milk	58.0	76
1 slice toasted Low Sodium Bread (See Menu 1)	3.5	97
1 t. Butter	0.2	38
Coffee—2 t. cream, 1 t. sugar	3.8	65
	69.6	424

LUNCH

	Milligrams Sodium	Calories
Rice and Tomato Soup	56.6	214
Mushroom Omelet*	73.8	727
2 oz. Lettuce and ½ Tomato	8.4	14
Apple Sauce-Supreme*	30.7	86
1 Slice Low Sodium Bread	3.5	97
1 L Butter	0.2	38
Coffee—2 t. cream, 1 t. sugar	3.8	65
	177	641

DINNER

	Milligrams Sodium	Calories
½ Grapefruit with 1 t. Honey	2.3	39
Beef Stew (2/3 of recipe for today, 1/3 for tomorrow lunch)*	151.4	386
1 Slice Low Sodium Bread	3.5	97
Endive Salad— ¼ Small Head	2.6	1
1 T. French Dressing (See Menu 3)		88
Apple Pie—1/8 slice*	2.9	388
Coffee with 1 t. sugar and 2 t. cream	3.8	65
	166.5	1064
Total for Day	413.1	2129

---

*Asterisks denote dishes for which recipes are given.

RECIPES FOR MENU 4

RICE AND TOMATO SOUP (Makes 2 plates)

	Milligrams Sodium	Calories
¼ cup rice (2⅔ ozs.)	4.8	272
½ cup tomatoes (unsalted)	20.4	24

	Milligrams Sodium	Calories
½ t. butter	0.1	19
¾ cup milk	87.8	114
	113.1	429
Portion for one	56.6	214

Boil up 4 cups of water. Wash rice and throw into boiling water. Boil until rice is soft, about 1 hour. Then boil tomatoes separately and rub them through strainer. Combine with rice. Add butter and milk and simmer a while.

MUSHROOM OMELET

	Milligrams Sodium	Calories
1 egg	67.0	77
1 t. butter	0.2	38
¼ onion (½ oz.)	1.4	4
1 T. green pepper (½ oz.)		4
2 oz. mushrooms	5.2	4
	73.8	127

Saute onion, mushrooms and green pepper in butter. When almost done add beaten egg and fry.

APPLE SAUCE SUPREME it making it in quantity large enough for 6 servings)

	Milligrams Sodium	Calories
8 t. milk	19.2	24
1/6 egg	11.3	13
1 t. sugar		19
1/3 cup apple sauce, canned (3 oz.)	0.2	30
few grains cinnamon		
10 drops vanilla extract		
nutmeg		
	30.7	86

Scald milk. Beat egg slightly. Add sugar, cinnamon to egg. Add hot milk to egg slowly, stirring constantly. Cook over hot water, stirring constantly until mixture coats a spoon. Remove. Add vanilla. Chill. Fold this sauce and apple sauce together. Serve in sherberts, sprinkled with nutmeg on top.

BEEF STEW
(Enough for dinner and lunch tomorrow)

	Milligrams Sodium	Calories
½ lb. beef	156.8	400
½ T. vegetable oil (Spry, Crisco)		55
1 potato	8.0	96
Bit of green pepper		
1 medium onion (2 oz.)	5.8	14
1 carrot (2 oz.)	54.0	12
1 T. juice from tomatoes (canned unsalted)	2.5	3
Few grains of pepper		
Few grains of sugar		
	227.1	580

2/3 for dinner equals 151.4 mg and 386 calories.

Cut beef in cubes. Dredge with peppered flour. Brown on all sides in vegetable oil. Quarter potato, mince green pepper, peel onions, scrape carrots and cut in fourths lengthwise. Add to meat with remaining ingredients. Simmer 2 hours or until meat is tender. Thicken gravy with flour if desired.

PASTRY FOR 2-CRUST PIES

	Milligrams Sodium	Calories
2 cups flour	5.4	900
¼ lb. butter	5.6	904
	11.0	1804

Sift flour. Cut in shortening until particles are the size of small peas. Sprinkle ½ T. cold water on mixture and mix in lightly with fork. Continue adding water in this fashion until the pastry gathers around the fork in a soft ball. Roll on lightly floured board to 1/8" thickness.

FILLING-APPLES

	Milligrams Sodium	Calories
1 lb. tart apples	9.6	60
1 cup sugar	0.8	896
2 t. flour	0.1	22
2 T. butter	1.4	226
Bit of nutmeg and cinnamon		
	11.09	1304

Quarter apples and slice thin. Line 9" pie pan with pastry. Mix sugar, flour and spices. Rub a little of this into pastry. Arrange apples and add remaining mixture. Dot with butter. Place top crust on. Make slits. Bake in hot oven 400° 45 min.

MENU 5
BREAKFAST

	Milligrams Sodium	Calories
8 oz. Pineapple Juice	2.2	144
1 cup Puffed Wheat (½ oz.)	0.4	55
½ Banana, cut in cereal (2 oz.)	0.4	26
½ cup Milk	58.0	76
1 Hot Roll	8.0	77
1 t. Butter	0.2	38
Coffee—2 t. cream and 1 t. sugar	3.8	65
	73.0	481

LUNCH

	Milligrams Sodium	Calories
Beef Stew left over from yesterday's meal (Menu 4)	76.0	193
1 Hot Roll	8.0	77
1 t. Butter	0.2	38
Salad: ½ orange, 2 oz. lettuce	8.0	22
4 oz. canned peaches (2 halves)	6.8	76
Coffee—2 t. cream, 1 t. sugar	3.8	65

	102.8	471

DINNER

	Milligrams Sodium	Calories
8 oz. Breaded Veal Cutlet*	240.8	488
4 oz. Pan-Fried Potatoes*	8.0	316
4 oz. Brussel Sprouts*	9.0	69
Salad: ½ cucumber, 2 oz. lettuce, ½ tomato, ¼ green pepper	8.8	22
Custard Cake Pudding*	34.5	317
	301.1	1212
Total for the Day	476.9	2164

RECIPES FOR MENU 5

ROLLS

	Milligrams Sodium	Calories
½ yeast cake (½ oz.)	0.5	12
½ cup milk	58.0	76
½ cup flour	1.3	225
½ egg	33.3	38
7 T. flour	1.4	231
2 T. sugar	0.1	112
2 T. melted butter	1.4	226
	96.0	920
This recipe makes 12 rolls. 1 roll equals	8.0	77

Scald milk, cool to lukewarm, and add to crumbled yeast cake. Stir until yeast is dissolved. Add flour. Let rise in warm place until light. Beat egg, stir into yeast mixture with sugar and shortening. Add enough flour to make stiff dough (about 7 T.) Spread with melted butter. Cover. Place in refrigerator overnight. Then rise until double. Roll thick on lightly covered board. Cut with biscuit cutter 2" in diameter. Spread with melted butter. Fold over. Cover, let rise until double. Bake in hot oven 10-12 min.

BREADED VEAL CUTLET

28

½ lb. veal cutlet
Bread crumbs
Beaten egg
Vegetable shortening
Total given by McCance and Widdowson   240.8   488

Wipe cutlets with damp cloth. Sprinkle with pepper. Dip in crumbs. Dip in beaten eggs and then in crumbs again. Saute slowly in melted fat until well-browned. Add some water, about 2 T. and cover. Simmer until thoroughly cooked.

BRUSSELS SPROUTS

	Milligrams Sodium	Calories
¼ lb. brussels sprouts	8.8	20
1 t. butter	0.2	38
1 t. flour		11
	9.0	69

Cook sprouts until tender. Then melt butter. Add flour and a little water from cooked sprouts. Pour over sprouts and serve.

PAN-FRIED POTATOES

	Milligrams Sodium	Calories
¼ lb. potatoes	8.0	96
2 T. vegetable shortening		220
	8.0	316

Slice potatoes thin. Soak in cold water for ½ hour. Dry. Heat oil and place slices in pan. Cover. Brown on both sides.

CUSTARD CAKE PUDDING

	Milligrams Sodium	Calories
¼ cup sugar	0.2	224
½ T. flour	0.1	16
¼ cup milk	0.2	38
¼ lemon	0.5	1
½ egg beaten separately	33.5	38

34.5   317

Mix sugar and flour. Add milk to egg yolks, pour over sugar mixture and mix well. Then add beaten whites and juice and grated rind of lemon. Put in buttered dish, set in pan of hot water and bake 40 min. in moderate oven. Turn out on serving dish when cold. Liquid in bottom of pan serves as sauce. You may serve with whipped cream.

MENU 6
BREAKFAST

	Milligrams Sodium	Calories
8 oz. Apricot Nectar	4.0	136
¼ cup Instant Ralston (1 oz.) with	0.2	110
½ cup Milk with	58.0	76
2 T. Raisins	7.5	35
1 t. Butter 2	0.2	38
1 slice Low Sodium Bread (See Menu 1)	3.5	97
Coffee—2 t. cream, 1 t. sugar	3.8	65
	77.2	557

LUNCH

	Milligrams Sodium	Calories
Spicy Creamed Egg*	106.5	225
1 Boiled Mashed Potato	4.0	92
Stewed Carrots*	55.8	91
Peach Cocktail*	6.0	99
Coffee—2 t. cream, 1 t. sugar	3.8	65
	176.1	572

DINNER

	Milligrams Sodium	Calories
Lamb Curry with Rice*	163.3	609
¼ lb. Green Peas, cooked		56
2 oz. Hearts of Lettuce	6.8	6

30

	Milligrams Sodium	Calories
4 t. Vinegar Dressing (see Menu 1)	3.0	63
Lemon Sponge Pudding*	53.8	226
Coffee—2 t. cream, 1 t. sugar	3.8	65
	230.7	1025
Total for the Day	484.0	2154

RECIPES FOR MENU 6
SPICY CREAMED EGGS (To be served with Mashed Potatoes)

	Milligrams Sodium	Calories
1 egg—hardboiled	67.0	77
1/3 cup milk	39.0	50
2 t. flour	0.1	22
Pinch of chilli powder		
Bit of minced onion		
	106.5	225

Add flour and chili to melted butter and blend. Add milk, minced onion. Cook over hot water stirring until thickened. Cut eggs in quarters and add. Serve with mashed potatoes.

STEWED CARROTS

	Milligrams Sodium	Calories
¼ medium onion (½ oz.)	1.4	3
2 t. butter	0.4	76
1 medium sliced carrot (2 oz.)	54.0	12
Pepper		
	55.8	91

Chop onion fine. Saute slowly in butter until tender. Add carrots and pepper. Cover and simmer over low heat for 30 min. Add some water if necessary.

PEACH COCKTAIL

	Milligrams Sodium	Calories

31

2 peaches (5 oz.)	4.0	55
½ T. honey	1.3	27
1 t. lemon juice		
3 T. orange juice	0.7	17
2/3 cup hot water		
	6.0	99

Peel and stone the peaches. Mash them. Add honey and water. Stir and allow to cool. Then add juices of lemon and oranges. Serve chilled in sherbert glasses.

LAMB CURRY

	Milligrams Sodium	Calories
5 oz. lean lamb (weighed without the bone)	157.0	265
½ onion, sliced thin (1 oz.)	1.5	3
2½ t. shortening (butter)	0.5	95
½ t. curry	0.5	3
1 T. flour	0.2	33
1 cup hot boiled rice (6 oz.)	3.6	210
	163.3	609

Cut lamb into small cubes, removing all fat Brown slightly. Brown onions until they are almost black and add to lamb. Add curry powder and boiling water, just enough to cover. Cover and simmer 2 hours or more until very tender. Add more water if necessary. When cooked, thicken sauce with flour. Have rice cooked very dry and serve the rice and curried lamb on top.

LEMON SPONGE PUDDING (This is a recipe for 2)

	Milligrams Sodium	Calories
1 egg, beaten separately	67.0	77
1/3 lemon rind and juice	1.7	4
1/3 cup sugar	0.2	298
2 t. flour	0.1	22
1/3 cup milk	38.6	50
	107.6	451

1 portion equals 53.8 mg. of sodium and 226 calories Add grated rind and juice to egg yolks which have been beaten until thick and lemon colored. Add mixture of sugar and flour slowly. Beat egg whites until stiff enough to hold their shape and fold into the mixture. Pour into shallow dish. Set in pan of cold water and bake 45 minutes in moderate oven.

MENU 7
BREAKFAST

	Milligrams Sodium	Calories
1 Orange, sliced	2.4	32
1 cup Puffed Rice (½ oz.) with	0.1	60
2 oz. Blueberries with	0.2	30
½ cup Milk	58.0	76
1 slice Low Sodium Bread (toasted) (See Menu 1)	3.5	97
1 t. Butter	0.2	38
1 T. Marmalade	5.2	74
Coffee—2 t. Cream and 1 t. Sugar	3.8	65
	3.8	65

LUNCH

	Milligrams Sodium	Calories
Curried Egg and Mushrooms	78.8	242
1 t. Butter	0.2	38
1 slice Low Sodium Bread	3.5	97
Vegetable salad: ½ tomato, 1 oz. lettuce, 1 oz. green pepper, 1 oz. cucumber	8.8	22
½ cup Milk	58.0	76
3 Seed Cookies*	12.0	255
	161.3	255

DINNER

	Milligrams Sodium	Calories

	Milligrams Sodium	Calories
½ lb. Pan-Browned Pork Chops with*	70.6	34
Sauce Creole (make 2 portions, one for tomorrow's lunch for the spaghetti)	5.0	20
1 Baked Sweet Potato (4 oz.)	20.4	92
2½ oz. Candied Carrots*	68.1	62
½ oz. Endive Salad (¼ small head) with	2.6	1
4 t. Vinegar Dressing (see Menu 1)	3.0	63
Marmalade Tapioca*	96.2	323
	265.9	865
Total for the Day	500.6	2067

----

*Asterisks denote dishes for which recipes are given.

RECIPES FOR MENU 7
CURRIED EGGS AND MUSHROOMS (Serve on Toast)

	Milligrams Sodium	Calories
¼ t. curry powder	0.2	1
2 T. cream	11.4	115
1 hard cooked egg, chopped	67.0	77
1 t. chopped onion		
1 t. butter	0.2	38
1 t. flour		11
¼ cup water		
	78.8	242

Cook onion and mushroom in fat until tender and slightly brown. Add flour and stir well. Add water gradually and cook until thick, stirring constantly. Add curry powder and simmer for 10 minutes. Add egg. Stir in cream and bring to boiling point. Serve at once on toast.

SEED CAKES Recipe makes 20 cookies

	Milligrams Sodium	Calories

	Milligrams Sodium	Calories
½ cup sugar	0.4	448
3/8 cup shortening, Spry, Crisco, or butter	4.2	678
1 egg slightly beaten	67.0	77
4 t. brandy	0.5	51
Grated rind of ½ lemon	1.7	4
1 cup flour	2.7	450
3 T. caraway seeds	3.0	
	79.5	1708

1 cookie equals 4.0 mg. of sodium and 85 calories.

Cream sugar and butter well. Add eggs, brandy, lemon rind, and flour. Roll thin. Sprinkle with seeds. Roll again and cut in fancy shapes. Bake 15 minutes in 300 degree oven.

PAN BROWNED PORK CHOPS AND CREOLE SAUCE

	Milligrams Sodium	Calories
½ lb. pork chops lean, weighed with bone	70.6	304
Creole sauce for 2:		
½ onion chopped fine, 1 oz	1.5	4
2 T. sweet red pepper, chopped fine	0.1	8
2 T. green peppers, chopped fine	0.1	8
½ T. parsley, 1/5 oz	1.8	1
Bit of garlic	0.5	1
2 mushrooms cut small, 1 oz.	2.6	2
1 tomato, peeled and cut	3.2	16
	9.8	40

Cook chops slowly for ½ hour. Add creole sauce. Put in baking dish and bake slowly for 1 hour to 1½ hours, basting at ½ hour intervals.

Sauce: Combine all ingredients and cook slowly for one hour.

CANDIED CARROTS

	Milligrams Sodium	Calories
2½ oz. carrots	68.0	15

	Milligrams Sodium	Calories
10 drops lemon juice		
½ T. sugar		28
2 t. water		
½ t. butter	0.1	19
	68.1	62

Clean carrots and cut lengthwise. Add all ingredients Cover and cook over low heat until tender and glazed.

MARMALADE TAPIOCA (Can best be made for 6 servings)

	Milligrams Sodium	Calories
1/6 egg	11.0	13
2/3 cup milk	77.3	101
1 T. tapioca	0.4	34
4 t. sugar		76
1/6 lemon	0.6	1
4 t. orange marmalade	6.9	98
	96.2	323

Mix egg yolk with small amount of the milk. Add tapioca* sugar, and rest of milk. Cook over rapidly boiling water 10-12 minutes, stirring frequently. Beat egg white stiff. Fold hot mixture into egg white. Cool. Fold in lemon juice and rind and add ½ cup orange marmalade. Serve in sherbert glasses.

MENU 8
BREAKFAST

	Milligrams Sodium	Calories
4 oz. Grapefruit Juice (unsweetened)	0.4	40
2 T. Farina 2/3 oz. (Do not use the quick cooking type)	0.1	67
½ cup Milk	58.0	76
1 sl. Cinnamon Toast. (Use low sodium bread—see Menu 1)	5.5	97
1 t. Butter	0.2	58

	5.8	65
Coffee—2 t. cream, 1 t. sugar	66.0	585

LUNCH

	Milligrams Sodium	Calories
1 Scrambled Egg	67.0	77
1 t. Butter	0.2	58
2 oz. Spaghetti with	4.4	64
Creole Sauce (made for pork chops on Menu 7)	5.0	20
Salad, 2 oz. lettuce and ½ sliced orange	8.0	22
2 Sugar Cookies	0.6	156
Coffee—2 t. cream, 1 t. sugar	5.8	65
	89.0	422

DINNER

	Milligrams Sodium	Calories
Spanish Chicken*	193.3	650
French Fried Onions*	70.5	502
1 Boiled Potato, sprinkled with Parsley	4.0	92
1 slice Low Sodium Bread	5.5	97
Salad: 1 oz. cabbage and 1 oz. pineapple	6.9	20
Spicy Baked Apple*	2.1	152
Coffee—2 t. cream, 1 t. sugar	5.8	65
	283.9	1558
Total for the day	458.9	2165

----

* Asterisks denote dishes for which recipes are given.

RECIPES FOR MENU 8
SUGAR COOKIES (Makes 2 dozen cookies)

	Milligrams Sodium	Calories
1 cup flour	27	450
¼ cup sugar	0.2	224
½ cup butter	5.6	904
1 T. sugar		56
½ t. vanilla extract		
	8.5	1634

1 cookie equals .3 mg. sodium and 68 calories

Mix flour and sugar. Rub in shortening with fingertips. Form into long rolls, wrap in waxed paper. Chill until firm. Slice thin, place on baking sheet.. Mix tablespoon sugar with vanilla. Sprinkle on cookies. Bake in moderately hot oven until slightly browned.

SPANISH CHICKEN

	Milligrams Sodium	Calories
¾ lb. frying chicken (weighed with bone)	146.4	348
7/8 cup canned tomatoes (unsalted) 7 oz	35.7	42
1/8 t. sugar		
¼ lb. mushrooms	10.4	8
½ cup cooked peas	0.4	56
2 T. flour and pepper	0.4	66
1 T. cooking oil (vegetable oils)		110
	193.3	630

Wipe chicken well and dredge in flour seasoned with pepper. Brown in small quantity of oil. Add tomatoes and sugar. Cover. Simmer ½ hour or until tender. Add cleaned mushrooms to chicken. Add cooked peas. Heat 10 minutes and serve.

FRENCH FRIED ONIONS

	Milligrams Sodium	Calories
2 medium onions, 4 oz.	11.6	28
½ cup milk	58.5	76
1½ T. salad oil		165
1 T. flour	0.2	33

70.3	302

Soak onion rings in milk about 10 minutes. Dip in flour and fry in heated fat until brown. Drain.

SPICY BAKED APPLE

	Milligrams Sodium	Calories
1 apple	2.0	40
4 t. water		
2 whole cloves		
2 T. sugar	0.1	112
Small bit of stick cinnamon		
	2.1	152

Wash and core apple. Place piece of cinnamon in center. Stick with cloves and place in pan. Add water, cover. Bake in moderate oven 30 minutes until tender but not soft. Remove. Combine liquid from pan with sugar. Boil 1 minute. Baste apples with syrup and place under to glaze tops.

MENU 9
BREAKFAST

	Milligrams Sodium	Calories
½ Grapefruit	0.8	12
¼ cup Maitex—Wheat Cereal, 1 oz	1.0	110
½ cup Milk	58.0	76
1 Hot Roll (see Menu 5)	8.0	77
1 t. Butter	0.2	38
Coffee—2 t. cream, 1 t sugar	3.8	65
	71.8	378

LUNCH

	Milligrams Sodium	Calories
Strained Vegetable Soup	62.3	133

	Milligrams Sodium	Calories
French Omelet*	67.2	115
Salad: 1 oz. cucumber, 1 oz. lettuce, ½ tomato	8.0	14
1 T. French Dressing (see Menu 3)		88
1 Roll and 1 t. Butter	8.2	115
Coffee—2 t. cream, 1 t. sugar	3.8	65
	149.5	530

DINNER

	Milligrams Sodium	Calories
Baked Cod in Milk*	229.7	394
1 Boiled Potato	4.0	92
Fried Eggplant*	5.8	138
1 Roll	8.0	77
Tropical Pudding*	9.0	245
Coffee—2 t. cream, 1 t. sugar	3.8	65
	260.3	1011
Total for the day	481.6	1919

---

* Asterisks denote dishes for which recipes are given.

RECIPES FOR MENU 9

STRAINED VEGETABLE SOUP (Makes 3 plates)

	Milligrams Sodium	Calories
1 carrot 2 oz	54.0	12
1 onion 2 oz.	5.8	14
1 potato 4 oz.	8.0	96
1 tomato 3 oz.	2.4	12
1 T. butter	0.7	113
1 cup milk	116.1	152
Pepper		
	187.0	399

1 plate equals 62.3 mg. of sodium and 133 calories.

Cut up vegetables. Put up in enough water to cover and boil until potato and carrot are soft. Then pour thru soup strainer and mash vegetables fine. Add butter, milk and pepper. Allow to simmer.

FRENCH OMELET

	Milligrams Sodium	Calories
1 t. butter	0.2	38
1 egg	67.0	77
1 T. water		
Pepper		
	67.2	115

Add water and pepper to well beaten egg. Pour into melted butter in frying pan and cook over low heat until the egg is done at bottom. Tilt and allow uncooked portions to flow to bottom. Repeat until egg is cooked thruout. Fold and serve.

BAKED COD IN MILK

	Milligrams Sodium	Calories
½ lb. cod	136.0	192
3 T. cream	17.1	172
3 T. water		
2 T. fine bread crumbs	76.6	30
Pepper		
Chopped chives or scallions as garnish		
	229.7	394

Place fish steaks in greased baking dish. Pre-heat oven to moderate temperature. Mix cream with water and pour over fish and bake uncovered for 25 minutes to half hour. Add bread crumbs and pepper, sprinkle over carefully. Return to oven until crumbs have absorbed some of the sauce. Serve with chipped chives or scallions as a garnish.

FRIED EGGPLANT

	Milligrams Sodium	Calories
8 oz. eggplant	5.6	52
2 t. vegetable shortening		75
Pepper		
1 T. flour	0.2	55
	5.8	158

Pare eggplant—cut in thin slices. Pepper. Dip in flour and cook slowly in oil until they turn brown on both sides.

TROPICAL PUDDING

	Milligrams Sodium	Calories
1/3 banana	0.4	22
5 T. canned pineapple 1 oz	0.3	18
5 T. sliced strawberries	1.0	10
1/3 cup cooked rice 2¼ oz	1.5	79
4 t. heavy cream	6.0	80
2 t. powdered sugar		56
1 whole strawberry		
	9.0	245

Cut banana, combine with pineapple and strawberries. Add fruits to rice. Whip cream, add powdered sugar, fold into rice and fruit mixture. Serve in glasses with whole strawberry.

MENU 10
BREAKFAST

	Milligrams Sodium	Calories
4 oz. Canned Pears (2 halves)	9.2	72
¼ cup Wheatena 1 oz	0.2	110
½ cup Milk (hot) spiced with	58.0	76
1 t. sugar and bit of cinnamon		19
1 Roll (see Menu 5)	8.0	77
2 t. Butter	0.4	76

| Coffee—2 t. cream, 1 t. sugar | 3.8 | 65 |
| | 79.6 | 495 |

LUNCH

	Milligrams Sodium	Calories
Sliced Hard Boiled Eggs on 2 oz. of Lettuce	73.8	83
Cucumbers in Sour Cream*	15.6	119
2 Sugar Cookies (see Menu 8)	0.6	136
Coffee—2 t. cream, 1 t. sugar	3.8	65
	93.8	403

DINNER

	Milligrams Sodium	Calories
8 oz. Steak, Broiled	156.8	400
1 Baked Potato and 1 t. Butter	8.2	134
¼ lb. Buttered String Beans, 1 t. Butter	3.8	46
Salad: ½ apple, ½ grapefruit slices on lettuce leaf	5.4	35
1 T. French Dressing (see Menu 3)		88
2½ oz. Ice Cream (1 gill)	71.2	145
Coffee—2 t. cream, 1 t. sugar	3.8	65
	249.2	913
Total for the day	422.6	1811

---

* Asterisks denote dishes for which recipes are given.

RECIPES FOR MENU 10

CUCUMBERS IN SOUR CREAM

	Milligrams Sodium	Calories
¼ medium cucumber	1.8	1
¼ medium onion	1.4	3

	Milligrams Sodium	Calories
2 T. sour cream	11.4	115
1 t. vinegar	1.0	
Bit of sugar, dry mustard, black pepper, garlic		
	15.6	119

Slice cucumber and onion thin. Rub dish with garlic. Place onion on bottom, cucumber on top, in layers. Cover mixture with remaining ingredients blended into a dressing. Cover and chill before serving.

MENUS 11-20

900- 1000 Milligrams of Sodium 1800 - 2200 Calories

MENU 11
BREAKFAST

	Milligrams Sodium	Calories
4 oz. Strawberries with	1.6	28
1 t. Sugar with		19
3 T. Sweet Cream	17.1	174
1 Poached Egg	67.0	77
1 slice Whole Wheat Bread (toasted)	123.0	70
1 t. Butter	0.2	38
Coffee—2 t. cream, 1 t. sugar	3.8	65
	212.7	471

LUNCH

	Milligrams Sodium	Calories
1 plate Strained Vegetable Soup (see Menu 9)	62.3	133
1 Lamb Chop, broiled (3¹/₃ oz.)	104.6	176
4 oz. Green Peas, buttered,	1 0.6	94

	Milligrams Sodium	Calories
t. Butter		
1 slice Whole Wheat Bread	123.0	70
2 oz. shredded Lettuce	6.8	6
1 T. French Dressing (see Menu 3)		88
Coffee—2 t. cream, 1 t. sugar	3.8	65
2 Tea Cookies	7.4	154
	308.5	786

DINNER

	Milligrams Sodium	Calories
½ lb. Breaded Veal Cutlets (see Menu 5)	240.8	488
Stewed Tomatoes*	73.2	129
1 Baked Potato	8.0	96
1 slice Whole Wheat Bread	123.0	70
Salad: ½ apple, ½ grapefruit slices on lettuce leaf	5.4	35
4 oz. Fruit Salad, canned	10.0	80
	460.4	898
Total for the day	981.6	2155

---

* Asterisk denote dishes for which recipes are given.

RECIPES FOR MENU 11

TEA COOKIES (Will make 10 Cookies)

	Milligrams Sodium	Calories
3 T. shortening, Spry, Crisco, or butter	2.1	339
3 T. sugar	0.1	168
½ egg	33.5	38
10 drops vanilla extract		
½ cup flour	1.4	225

	37.1	770
1 Cookie equals	3.7	77

STEWED TOMATOES

	Milligrams Sodium	Calories
1 T. minced onion ½ oz	1.4	3
1 t. butter	0.2	38
½ cup tomatoes, canned, unsalted	20.4	24
4 t. bread crumbs	51.0	20
1 t. browned butter	0.2	38
Bit of bay leaf		
Bit of pepper		
1/3 t. sugar		6
½ clove		
	73.2	129

Chop onion fine. Cook in butter until slightly browned. Add tomatoes, bay leaf, pepper, sugar and cloves. Cover. Cook 10 minutes. Remove bay leaf and cloves. Toss bread crumbs in browned butter. Add to tomatoes; mix well.

MENU 12
BREAKFAST

	Milligrams Sodium	Calories
4 oz. Stewed Prunes (4 prunes)	3.4	120
¼ cup Oatmeal (1 oz.)	9.5	115
½ cup Milk	58.0	76
1 slice Whole Wheat Toast	123.0	70
1 t. Butter	0.2	38
1 T. Orange Marmalade	5.2	74
Coffee—2 t. cream, 1 t. sugar	3.8	65
	203.1	558

LUNCH

	Milligrams Sodium	Calories
Spring Vegetable Soup	20.0	106
Mushroom Omelet (see Menu 4)	73.8	127
1 slice Whole Wheat Bread	123.0	70
1 t. Butter	0.2	38
2 Tea Cookies (see Menu 11)	7.4	154
Coffee—2 t. cream, 1 t. sugar	3.8	65
	228.2	560

DINNER

	Milligrams Sodium	Calories
½ Grapefruit and 1 t. Honey	2.3	39
Macaroni with Liver*	79.6	231
Stewed Carrots (see Menu 6)	55.8	91
1 slice Whole Wheat Bread	123.0	70
1 t. Butter	0.2	38
3 oz. Celery Hearts (about 2)	116.7	9
2½ oz. Ice Cream (1 gill)	71.2	145
2 Tea Cookies (see Menu 11)	7.4	154
Coffee—2 t. cream, 1 t. sugar	3.8	65
	460.0	842
Total for the day	891.3	1960

------

* Asterisks denote dishes for which recipes are given.

RECIPES FOR MENU 12

SPRING VEGETABLE SOUP

	Milligrams Sodium	Calories
1 leek (¼ oz.)	2.5	2
1/3 cup shelled peas (1²/₃ oz.)	0.4	30
1/3 cup asparagus tips, raw (2 oz.)	1.0	10
1/3 pint water		
½ T. butter	0.3	57

	Milligrams Sodium	Calories
3 T. string beans (1 oz.)	1.8	4
1/6 carrot (½ oz.)	14.0	3
Pepper		
	20.0	106

Heat butter in pot. Add white part of leek cut up small, peas, carrots cut up small, asparagus tips cut up, and finely cubed string beans. Simmer gently 5 minutes covered. Then add water and pepper and cook 20 minutes.

MACARONI AND LIVER

	Milligrams Sodium	Calories
2 oz. elbow macaroni	4.4	64
3 oz. sliced liver	73.2	123
1 t shortening (butter)	0.2	38
Bit of chopped onion	0.2	38
Bit of crushed garlic	0.2	
2 t. boiling water		
Slice of tomato, diced (1 oz.)	0.8	4
	79.6	231

Dice liver. Heat fat in heavy skillet and put in liver, onion and garlic. Saute until tender and brown. Add tomato and pepper and boiling water and cook ten minutes. Have macaroni freshly boiled and drained. Turn into hot serving dish, add liver, mix well, and serve at once.

MENU 13
BREAKFAST

	Milligrams Sodium	Calories
8 oz. Orange Juice	4.0	88
Puffy Omelet	69.0	114
1 slice Whole Wheat Toast	123.0	70
1 t. Butter	0.2	38
Coffee—2 t. cream, 1 t. sugar	3.8	65
	200.0	375

48

LUNCH

	Milligrams Sodium	Calories
4 oz. Sauteed Mushrooms on*	16.6	98
1 slice Whole Wheat Toast	123.0	70
1 t. Butter	0.2	38
Salad: ½ orange and 2 oz. lettuce	8.0	22
2 Macaroons*	53.03	289
Coffee—2 t. cream, 1 t. sugar	3.8	65
	204.9	582

DINNER

	Milligrams Sodium	Calories
Meat Loaf*	255.1	297
1 Boiled Parsley Potato	4.0	92
Peas and Com with Curry*	246.5	143
Apple Salad and*	14.6	88
1 T. French Dressing (see Menu 3)		88
Fruit Cup with Wine*	5.7	125
Coffee—2 t. cream, 1 t. sugar	3.8	65
	529.7	898
Total for the day	934.6	1855

RECIPES FOR MENU 13

PUFFY OMELET

	Milligrams Sodium	Calories
1 egg white—1 egg yolk	67.0	77
1 T. water		
Few grains paprika	2.0	
Few grains pepper		
1 t. salad oil		37
	69.0	114

Add water, paprika, pepper to beaten egg yolks. Beat egg whites. Fold yolks into egg whites lightly. Heat salad oil in pan until all pan is coated.

Pour mixture into pan and spread evenly. Cook over low heat until omelet is puffed and brown on bottom. Then set in moderate oven 5 minutes until top is firm to touch. Fold and turn on hot plate.

MUSHROOMS SAUTEED

	Milligrams Sodium	Calories
4 oz. mushrooms	10.4	8
1 small onion	5.8	14
2 t. butter	0.4	76
	16.6	98

Cut up an onion and saute in butter. Place washed and cut up mushrooms into onion when it is light brown. Allow to simmer. Pepper it. Serve on toast.

MACAROONS (Suggest making about 4 times the recipe)

	Milligrams Sodium	Calories
4 t. sweetened condensed milk (1-1/9 oz,)		
1/3 cup moist coconut (1 oz.)		
5 drops vanilla extract		
3 drops almond extract		
	53.3	289

Makes 2 macaroons.

Combine condensed milk and shredded coconut. Add vanilla and almond extracts. Drop by spoonfuls on greased baking sheet Bake in moderate oven 10 minutes or until brown.

MEAT LOAF

	Milligrams Sodium	Calories
½ cup tomatoes, canned, unsalted (4 oz.)	20.4	24
4 oz. ground beef	78.4	200
¼ cup bread crumbs	143.7	56
1/6 egg	11.1	13
1 T. onion (½ oz.)	1.5	4

Drain tomatoes. Add pulp to ground meat. Add crumbs and pepper. Beat egg. Add. Mince onion and add. Mix thoroughly. Grease pan and pack meat in. Bake in hot oven 45 minutes.

PEAS AND CORN WITH CURRY

	Milligrams Sodium	Calories
1/3 cup canned drained green peas (2 oz.)	132.0	48
¼ cup whole kernel corn, canned (2 oz.)	114.2	38
½ T. butter	0.3	57
Bit of curry powder		
	246.5	143

Combine peas and corn. Melt butter and add curry powder. Pour over vegetables and mix well. Heat and serve.

APPLE SALAD

	Milligrams Sodium	Calories
½ cup crushed canned pineapple (3 oz.)	0.8	54
½ cup shredded cabbage (2 oz.)	12.8	14
apple chopped	1.0	20
	14.6	88

Drain syrup from pineapple. Mix pineapple, cabbage and apple. Add dressing.

FRUIT CUP WITH WINE

	Milligrams Sodium	Calories
1 cubed orange	2.4	32
1 cubed banana (small)	0.8	52
2 T. pineapple bits		11
Seeded grapes (1 oz.)	1.1	18
Flavor with Grenadine (½ oz.)	1.4	12
	5.7	125

Combine, chill, and serve.

MENU 14
BREAKFAST

	Milligrams Sodium	Calories
½ Grapefruit, sliced (4 oz.)	0.8	12
1 oz. Shredded Wheat—1 biscuit with	4.7	103
½ Banana (3 oz.)	0.6	39
½ cup Milk	58.0	76
1 T. Marmalade	5.2	74
Coffee—2 t. cream, 1 t. sugar	3.8	65
	73.1	369

LUNCH

	Milligrams Sodium	Calories
Baked Eggs in Sour Cream*	127.0	362
Salad: ½ apple, ½ grapefruit on lettuce	5.4	35
Slice Whole Wheat Bread	123.0	70
1 t. Butter	0.2	38
Coffee—2 t. cream, 1 t. sugar	3.8	65
	259.4	570

DINNER

	Milligrams Sodium	Calories
Baked Chicken (½ lb.)	216.7	509
Green Beans Creole (frozen)*	216.9	163
1 Mashed Potato	4.0	92
2 oz. Hearts of Lettuce	6.8	6
Early American Pudding*	102.3	264
Coffee—2 t. cream and 1 t. sugar	3.8	65
	550.5	1099
Total for the day	883.0	2038

RECIPES FOR MENU 14

BAKED EGGS IN SOUR CREAM

	Milligrams Sodium	Calories
3 T. chopped onions (1½ oz.)	4.3	11
½ T. shortening (butter)	0.3	57
1 egg	67.0	77
3 T. sour cream	17.1	172
1 T. buttered soft crumbs	38.3	45
	127.0	362

Cook onion until tender in butter. Spread this mixture on bottom of shallow, well-buttered casserole. Drop eggs on top of this and sprinkle with pepper. Bake in moderate oven 5 minutes. Remove and spread sour cream over eggs gently. Sprinkle with buttered crumbs. Return to oven for 10 minutes longer or until eggs are of the desired firmness.

BAKED CHICKEN

	Milligrams Sodium	Calories
½ lb. breast meat (not weighed with rest of chicken)	177.6	368
Bit of pepper		
1 T. flour	0.2	33
cup milk	38.6	51
½ T. butter	0.3	57
	216.7	509

Wash and dry chicken. Dust with peppered flour and place in roaster. Pour milk into roaster. Dot chicken with butter. Bake in hot oven 15 minutes. Reduce heat and bake for an hour longer. Baste chicken occasionally with milk in pan.

GREEN BEANS CREOLE

	Milligrams	Calories

	Sodium	
1 T. onion	1.4	4
1 t. salad oil		37
1/3 cup bread crumbs	191.4	75
½ cup canned tomatoes (4¹/₃ oz.)	22.1	26
½ cup frozen green beans (3-1/6 oz.)	2.0	21
Pepper		
	216.9	163

Saute onion in oil. Add bread crumbs. Then combine tomatoes, sugar and pepper. Cook green beans. Add liquid to tomatoes and cook until liquid is evaporated. Add green beans and place ½ mixture in bottom of casserole. Add ½ bread crumbs. Repeat and bake in hot oven.

EARLY AMERICAN PUDDING

	Milligrams Sodium	Calories
1 T. yellow com meal (½ oz.)		55
2/3 cup milk	77.0	101
4 t. molasses (1-1/9 oz.)	25.3	89
½ t. butter		19
Bit of ginger		
Bit of cinnamon		
	102.3	264

Combine cornmeal and spices. Scald half the milk, add slowly, stirring constantly. Add molasses. Mix thoroughly. Add remaining cold milk. Stir well. Cook over hot water, stirring occasionally, until slightly thickened. Pour into greased baking dish. Dot with butter. Set in pan of warm water and bake in slow oven about 2 hours.

MENU 15
BREAKFAST

	Milligrams Sodium	Calories
Baked Apple with 1 t. Sugar and Cinnamon	2.4	59

2 t. Cream	3.8	38
1 Boiled Egg	67.0	77
1 slice Whole Wheat Toast	123.0	70
1 t Butter	0.2	38
Coffee—2 t. cream and 1 t. sugar	3.8	65
	200.2	347

LUNCH

	Milligrams Sodium	Calories
½ Grapefruit (4 oz.) with 1 t. Honey	2.3	39
Vegetable Plate	17.2	277
1 slice Whole Wheat Bread	123.0	70
1 t. Butter	0.2	38
Chocolate Custard*	132.4	179
Coffee—2 t. cream and 1 t. sugar	3.8	65
	278.9	668

DINNER

	Milligrams Sodium	Calories
Broiled Flounder*	118.0	159
1 Baker Potato with	8.0	96
1 t. Butter	0.2	38
Scalloped Spinach*	188.0	108
Stuffed Celery*	112.7	25
Sweet Pilau*	25.8	501
Coffee—2 t. cream and 1 t. sugar	3.8	65
	456.5	992
Total for the day	935.6	2007

____
* Asterisks denote dishes for which recipes are given.

RECIPES FOR MENU 15

VEGETABLE PLATE

	Milligrams Sodium	Calories
1 potato (4 oz.)	8.0	96
1 oz. mushrooms	5.2	4
2 oz. yellow turnips	2.8	28
2 oz. green peas	0.5	36
1 T. butter	0.7	113
	17.2	277

Bake potato, saute mushrooms, boil mashed yellow turnips, and cook green peas. Serve.

CHOCOLATE CUSTARD (Recipe for 2)

	Milligrams Sodium	Calories
1/3 oz. unsweetened chocolate	0.3	60
1/3 cup strong coffee		
1/3 cup milk	39.0	51
½ egg	34.0	39
5 t. sugar		95
1 t. melted butter	0.2	38
10 drops vanilla extract		
1/3 cup bread crumbs	191.4	75
	264.9	358
For one portion	152.4	179

Melt chocolate over hot water. Add milk and strong coffee. Bring to a scalding point. Beat egg and add sugar. Pour milk mixture on egg mixture. Add melted butter and vanilla. Place crumbs in casserole and pour custard mixture on them. Set in fan of warm water. Bake in moderate oven until done, about hour.

BROILED FLOUNDER

	Milligrams Sodium	Calories
½ lb. of flounder (weighed with bone and skin)	117.6	120
Pepper		
Lemon juice (½ oz.)	0.2	1

	Milligrams Sodium	Calories
1 t. melted butter	0.2	38
	118.0	159

Split, clean and dry the fish. Sprinkle with pepper and lemon juice. Place skin side down on greased broiler. Broil 10 minutes, then turn and brown skin. Serve with melted butter flavored with lemon juice.

SCALLOPED SPINACH

	Milligrams Sodium	Calories
1/3 cup chopped cooked spinach (5-1/3 oz.)	116.3	25
1 t. minced onion		
Pepper		
1/6 egg	11.1	13
4 t. milk	9.6	12
4 t. buttered bread crumbs (38 cal. For butter)	51.0	58
	188.0	108

Combine spinach, onion and pepper. Beat egg slightly, combine with milk. Add to spinach. Top with buttered crumbs. Bake in oven until crumbs are brown.

STUFFED CELERY

	Milligrams Sodium	Calories
2 outer sulks of celery ($1^1/_3$ oz.— about 7" sulk)	51.8	4
4 t. cottage cheese	60.9	21
Bit of minced onion		
Bit of chili		
	112.7	25

Stuff celery sulk with cottage cheese and onion mixture. Sprinkle with bit of chili. Cut each stalk in small pieces and serve.

SWEET PILAU

	Milligrams Sodium	Calories

1 T. rice	1.2	68
½ T. butter	0.3	57
6 T. pineapple juice	0.3	54
2 t. brown sugar	1.5	23
1 T. seedless raisins	5.0	23
1 T. chopped walnuts	0.4	104
3 T. cream	17.1	172
	25.8	501

MENU 16
BREAKFAST

	Milligrams Sodium	Calories
8 oz. Orange and Grapefruit Juice	2.4	84
1 cup Puffed Rice (½ oz.) with	0.1	60
½ cup Milk with	58.0	76
2 T. Berries (Blueberries)	0.1	15
1 slice Whole Wheat Toast	123.0	70
1 t. Butter	0.2	38
Coffee—2 t cream and 1 t. sugar	3.8	65
	187.	408

LUNCH

	Milligrams Sodium	Calories
Asparagus Omelet*	68.1	87
1 Boiled Potato	4.0	92
1 t. Butter	0.2	38
Salad: 1 oz. cucumber, ½ tomato, 1 leaf lettuce	8.7	14
Pineapple and Cocoanut Dessert (see Menu 3)	3.4	123
1 slice Whole Wheat Bread	123.0	70
Coffee—2 t. cream and 1 t. sugar	3.8	65
	211.2	489

DINNER

	Milligrams	Calories

	Sodium	
½ Grapefruit with 1 t. Honey	2.3	39
8 oz. Broiled Sirloin Steak	156.8	400
French Fried Potatoes (made with one potato and fried in 2 T. vegetable oil)	8.0	316
Carrot Surprise*	300.7	93
Salad: 1 oz. green pepper, 1 oz. cucumber, ½ tomato and 1 leaf lettuce	8.3	22
Frozen Sherbert*	31.0	199
Coffee—2 t. cream and 1 t. sugar	3.8	65
	510.9	1134
Total for the day	909.7	2031

---

* Asterisks denote dishes for which recipes are given.

RECIPES FOR MENU 16
ASPARAGUS OMELET

	Milligrams Sodium	Calories
1 egg yolk—1 egg white	67.0	77
2 oz. cooked fresh asparagus	1.0	10
Dash of pepper		
Dash of paprika		
	68.0	87

Beat egg yolks. Add asparagus, pepper, paprika and mix. Beat whites stiff and fold in. Cook in hot greased frying pan on low heat until bottom is browned. Place in moderate oven a few minutes to dry out top. Cut omelet part way thru center, fold over and serve.

CARROT SURPRISE

	Milligrams Sodium	Calories
2/3 can diced carrots (3⅓ oz.)	267.0	17
½ egg	33.5	38
1 t. melted butter	0.2	38

Pepper

| | 300.7 | 93 |

Heat carrots, drain and mash. Beat egg. Add to carrots with pepper and butter. Pack in muffin pan. Set in pan of hot water and bake in moderate oven 20 minutes.

FROZEN SHERBERT (Recipe for 6)

	Milligrams Sodium	Calories
1 egg	67.0	77
1 cup sugar	0.8	896
1 cup milk	116.0	152
1 T. lemon juice	0.2	1
3 T. orange juice	0.7	17
4 oz. banana, mashed	0.8	52
	185.5	1195
Portion for one	31.0	199

Beat egg. Add sugar and milk. Then add the mashed bananas and orange and lemon juice. Freeze in refrigerator tray until mushy. At that point beat with a fork until creamy and smooth. Return to tray and refrigerate until ready to serve.

MENU 17
BREAKFAST

	Milligrams Sodium	Calories
8 oz. Pineapple Juice	0.8	144
¼ cup Wheatena (1 oz.)	0.2	110
½ cup Milk with	58.0	76
2 Stewed Prunes	1.7	60
1 slice Whole Wheat Toast	123.0	70
1 t. Butter	0.2	38
Coffee—2 t. cream and 1 t. sugar	3.8	65
	187.7	563

LUNCH

	Milligrams Sodium	Calories
Salmon Salad	277.1	134
1 Boiled Potato	4.0	92
1 slice Whole Wheat Bread	123.0	70
1 t. Butter	0.2	38
Cantaloupe Gelatin Salad* with	17.4	73
French Dressing for Fruit Salad*	1.0	134
Coffee—2 t. cream and 1 t. sugar	3.8	65
	426.56	606

DINNER

	Milligrams Sodium	Calories
Braised Veal Chops (shoulder)*	244.9	315
French Fried Bermuda Onions*	20.6	208
1 Boiled Potato	4.0	92
Orange Raisin Slaw*	20.2	56
Apple Pie—14 piece (see Menu 4)	2.9	388
Coffee—2 t. cream and 1 t. sugar	3.8	65
	296.4	1124
Total for the day	910.6	2293

---

* Asterisks denote dishes for which recipes are given.

RECIPES FOR MENU 17

SALMON SALAD

	Milligrams Sodium	Calories
2 oz. salmon, canned	268.4	120
1 small onion (1½ oz.)	4.3	11
1 t. vinegar	1.0	
1 large leaf lettuce	3.4	3
	277.1	134

Mix ingredients and serve on lettuce leaf.

CANTALOUPE GELATIN SALAD

	Milligrams Sodium	Calories
½ t unflavored gelatine		5
½ t. cold water		
1 t. boiling water		
1/3 cup ginger ale (2½ oz.)	4.0	28
1 t. sugar		19
½ cup cantaloupe balls (3 oz.)	11.0	21
Chicory		
	17.4	73

Sprinkle gelatin in cold water. Add boiling water, stir until dissolved. Add ginger ale and sugar. Chill until syrupy. Fold in cantaloupe balls. Pour into mold which has been chilled. Chill until firm. Garnish with chicory.

FRENCH DRESSING FOR FRUIT SALADS

	Milligrams Sodium	Calories
1 t. vinegar	1.0	
Pinch mustard		
½ t. sugar		3
2¼ t vegetable oil (olive oil)		131
¼ t. honey		
	1.0	134

BRAISED VEAL CHOPS

	Milligrams Sodium	Calories
8 oz. veal shoulder chops	243.2	248
1 t. butter	0.2	38
½ T. flour	0.1	17
1 T. sherry	1.4	12
¼ clove garlic, sliced		
	244.9	315

Wipe chops with clean damp cloth and dip in flour. Heat fat, brown chops quickly on both sides. Pour sherry or vinegar mixture over them. Place slivered garlic on top. Cover and simmer for 25 to 30 minutes, depending on thickness of chops. When serving, spoon liquid of pan over the chops.

FRENCH FRIED ONIONS

	Milligrams Sodium	Calories
½ large Bermuda onion (2 oz.)— cut thick slices	5.8	14
2 T. milk	14.4	18
2 T. flour	0.4	66
1 T. vegetable oil		110
	20.6	208

Separate rings. Soak in milk for 30 minutes. Dip in peppered flour and fry in hot fat.

ORANGE RAISIN SLAW

	Milligrams Sodium	Calories
1/3 orange	0.8	11
½ cup shredded cabbage (2 oz.)	12.8	14
1¹/₃ T. raisins, seedless	6.6	31
	20.2	56

Combine peeled oranges sliced, and shredded cabbage with raisins. French dressing may be added.

MENU 18
BREAKFAST

	Milligrams Sodium	Calories
1 Orange, sliced	2.4	32
Poached Egg in Cream	72.7	134
1 slice Whole Wheat Toast	123.0	70
1 t Butter	0.2	38
Coffee—2 t. cream and 1 t. sugar	3.8	65
	202.1	339

LUNCH

	Milligrams Sodium	Calories
4 oz. Grapefruit Juice	0.4	40
Tuna Potatoes, au Gratin*	323.8	334
2 oz. Shredded Lettuce	6.8	6
1 T. French Dressing (see Menu 3)		88
Banana and Grape Gelatin*	2.4	106
Coffee—2 t. cream and 1 t. sugar	3.8	65
	337.2	639

DINNER

	Milligrams Sodium	Calories
Erin Stew*	263.7	425
Salad: ½ cucumber, 1 tomato and 2 oz. lettuce	8.7	14
1 T. French Dressing (see Menu 3)		88
4 oz. Boiled String Beans with 1 t. Butter	3.8	46
Orange Rice Custard (see Menu 1)	30.6	409
Coffee—2 L cream and 1 t. sugar	3.8	65
	310.6	1047
Total for the day	849.9	2025

---

* Asterisks denote dishes for which recipes are given.

RECIPES FOR MENU 18

POACHED EGGS AND CREAM

	Milligrams Sodium	Calories
1 egg	67.0	77

1 T. heavy cream	5.7	57
	72.7	134

Butter pan generously. Set over low heat. Put cream in pan, break egg and slip into pan. Move pan slowly with circular motion until eggs are set.

TUNA AND POTATOES, AU GRATIN

	Milligrams Sodium	Calories
1 hot baked potato (4 oz.)	8.0	96
Bit of grated onion		
1½ oz. canned tuna (¼ cup)	231.3	131
½ oz. grated American cheddar	77.1	60
1 T. milk	7.2	9
1 t. butter	0.2	38
Pepper		
	323.8	334

Scoop out baked potatoes and mash. Season with milk, pepper and butter. Add grated onion. Drain and flake tuna and add. Refill potatoes. Sprinkle tops with cheese. Bake in moderate oven about 15 minutes.

BANANA AND GRAPE MOLD

	Milligrams Sodium	Calories
1 t. gelatin (plain)	0.7	10
1 T. cold water		
¼ cup grape juice (2 oz.)	0.5	36
½ T. sugar		28
t. lemon juice		
3 T. banana slices	0.3	20
3 T. diced oranges	0.9	12
	2.4	106

Sprinkle gelatin on cold water. Heat grape juice and pour over gelatin. Add sugar and lemon juice. Stir until dissolved. Chill until it thickens. Fold in the fruit and chill until firm.

ERIN STEW

	Milligrams Sodium	Calories
5 oz. top round beef	98.0	250
1 t. vegetable shortening		37
2 small onions (2½ oz.)	7.2	18
1 small carrot (2 oz.)	54.0	12
1 small potato (3 oz.)	6.0	72
1/3 cup canned peas (1½ oz.)	98.5	36
	263.7	425

Cut meat into cubes. Dredge in flour. Brown on all sides in fat. Peel onions. Add. Cut carrots in strips. Add. Cube potatoes and add. Simmer 2½ hours, adding water if necessary. Add peas, liquid and all. Simmer ½ hour longer.

MENU 19
BREAKFAST

	Milligrams Sodium	Calories
4 oz. Stewed Prunes (4 prunes)	3.4	120
¼ cup Maltex Cereal (1 oz.) with	1.1	110
½ cup Milk with	58.0	76
1 T. Raisins (¼ oz.)	5.0	23
1 slice Whole Wheat Bread	123.0	70
1 t. Butter	0.2	38
Coffee—2 t. cream and 1 t. sugar	3.8	65
	194.5	502

LUNCH

	Milligrams Sodium	Calories
Spring Salad*	204.03	226
1 slice Whole Wheat Bead	123.0	70
1 t. Butter	0.2	38
Apple Pudding*	160.9	379
Coffee—2 t. cream and 1 t. sugar	3.8	65
	492.2	778

DINNER

	Milligrams Sodium	Calories
Cod—Sweet and Sour*	213.5	171
1 Baked Potato	8.0	96
4 oz. Asparagus, boiled	2.0	20
Salad:Endive (1 oz.)	5.1	3
1 T. French Dressing (see Menu 3)		88
Coffee Mousse*	31.4	406
	260.0	784
Total for the day	946.7	2064

------

* Asterisks denote dishes for which recipes are given.

SPRING SALAD

	Milligrams Sodium	Calories
½ oz. lemon gelatin	47.0	60
cup water		
3 T. diced cucumber	5.5	5
3 T. sliced radishes	25.2	6
1 T. sliced scallions (½ oz.)	1.4	3
½ cup watercress (2/3 oz.)	11.0	2
1 T. mayonnaise	114.2	150
	204.3	226

Dissolve gelatin as directed on package. Add vinegar. Chill until syrupy. Fold in cucumber, radishes and scallions. Serve on watercress with mayonnaise.

APPLE PUDDING

	Milligrams Sodium	Calories
2 t. butter	0.4	76
1/3 cup apple sauce	0.1	30
¼ cup brown sugar (1¹/₃oz.)	9.1	140
¼ cup dry bread crumbs	143.7	56
4 t. heavy cream	7.6	77

Bit of vanilla extract

160.9	379

Melt butter, add apple sauce and sugar. Stir over low heat until browned. Remove. Add vanilla. Chill. Fill sherbert glasses with alternate layers of crumbs and apple sauce mixture. Begin and end with crumbs. Whip cream and place on top.

COD - SWEET AND SOUR

	Milligrams Sodium	Calories
½ lb. cod, weighed with bones and skin	184.0	152
½ onion (1 oz.)	1.5	3
½ carrot (1 oz.)	27.0	6
Bit of lemon		
½ t. sugar		10
All spice	1.0	
	213.5	171

Slice the onion and carrot and place in pot with enough water to cover. Cook about 15 minutes. Then cut in lemon, sugar and a little all spice and place the fish in the pot. Cook for 20 minutes on medium flame after cooking starts.

COFFEE MOUSSE

	Milligrams Sodium	Calories
½ t. unflavored gelatin		5
2 t. cold water		
4 t. strong brewed coffee	1.0	
1/3 cup heavy cream	30.4	306
5 t. powdered sugar		95
10 drops vanilla extract		
	31.4	406

Sprinkle gelatin on cold water. Dissolve in hot coffee. Chill until syrupy. Whip cream slightly. Add sugar, vanilla. Fold into coffee mixture. Freeze in tray.

MENU 20
BREAKFAST

	Milligrams Sodium	Calories
2 oz. Kadota Figs (2 figs)	0.5	100
Puffy Omelet (see Menu 13)	69.0	114
1 slice Whole Wheat Toast	123.0	70
1 t. Butter	0.2	38
Coffee—2 t. cream and 1 t. sugar	3.8	65
	196.5	387

LUNCH

	Milligrams Sodium	Calories
4 oz. Orange Juice	2.0	44
Salmon Salad	402.1	275
1 Boiled Potato	4.0	92
2 Tea Cookies (see Menu 2)	7.4	154
Coffee—2 t. cream and 1 t. sugar	3.8	65
	419.3	630

DINNER

	Milligrams Sodium	Calories
Pan Broiled Pork Chops with Apple*	73.0	377
Baked Sweet Potato	20.4	92
Spinach*	117.0	137
Hearts of Lettuce (2 oz.)	6.8	6
Baked Custard*	105.6	203
Coffee—2 t. cream and 1 t. sugar	3.8	65
2 Tea Cookies (see Menu 11)	7.4	154
	334.0	1034
Total for the day	949.8	

RECIPES FOR MENU 20

SALMON SALAD

	Milligrams Sodium	Calories
2 oz. salmon (about 5 T.)	268.4	120
1 T. diced celery (½ oz.)	19.5	1
t. minced green pepper		4
1 T. mayonnaise	114.2	150
	402.1	275

Bone the salmon and flake. Combine with celery, green pepper and mayonnaise. Serve on lettuce.

PAN BROILED PORK CHOPS WITH APPLE

	Milligrams Sodium	Calories
½ lb. pork chops, lean, weighed with bone	74.0	304
Pepper		
1 T. flour	0.2	33
1 apple	2.4	40
	73.0	377

Wipe chops and sprinkle with pepper, dust lightly with flour. Place in hot heavy frying pan, fat edge down. Brown on both sides. Pour off fat, cover and cook slowly until tender (about 25 minutes). Core and pare apple. Cut in ½ inch slices. Fry in fat remaining in pan and serve with chops.

SPINACH

	Milligrams Sodium	Calories
1 t. minced onion		
1 T. butter	0.7	113
½ cup hot chopped spinach (3⅓	116.3	24

oz.)

Pepper

	117.0	137

Saute onion in butter, pour over spinach, and add pepper. Mix thoroughly.

BAKED CUSTARD

	Milligrams Sodium	Calories
1 egg	67.0	77
1⅓ T. sugar		75
1/3 cup milk	38.6	51
1/6 t. vanilla		
Nutmeg		
	105.6	203

Beat eggs slightly. Add sugar, mix well. Scald milk. Add slowly, stirring constantly. Add vanilla extract. Pour into baking dish. Sprinkle with nutmeg. Set in pan of cold water. Bake in moderate oven 1¼ hours.

INTRODUCTION TO WEIGHT REDUCING MENUS

WEIGHT REDUCING MEALS
400 - 500 Milligrams of Sodium Below 1200 Calories

A portion of the weight of the obese person consists of water bound to sodium in his tissues. This excess water may be liberated and excreted during the maintenance of the low- sodium diet. In addition, the low-sodium diet tends to decrease the hydrochloric acid production in the stomach thereby decreasing hunger. The low-sodium diets for reducing which follow will be found to be of inestimable help in the program of weight reduction.

MENUS 21-30

MENU 21
BREAKFAST

	Milligrams Sodium	Calories
4 oz. Orange Juice (½ cup)	2.0	44
¼ cup Oatmeal (1 oz.)	9.5	115
½ cup Milk	58.0	76
Coffee (no sugar or cream)		8
1 slice Low Sodium Bread (see Menu 1)	3.5	97
	73.0	340

LUNCH

	Milligrams Sodium	Calories
Scrambled Egg and Mushrooms (see Menu 1)	81.1	130
Salad: ½ Grapefruit, 1 oz. Lettuce	4.2	15
Cherry and Banana Gelatin	47.6	123
Coffee (no sugar or cream)		8
	132.9	276

DINNER

	Milligrams Sodium	Calories
½ lb. Broiled Liver	195.2	328
4 oz. Mashed Yellow Turnips	5.6	56
Eggplant Mexican*	23.2	40
Salad: 2 oz. lettuce and 1 medium tomato	10.0	22
Vinegar Dressing—4 t.	3.0	19
Baked Apple with	2.4	40
1 t. Sugar and Cinnamon		19
Coffee	4.8	33
	244.2	557
Total for the day	450.1	1173

* Asterisks denote dishes for which recipes are given.

INTRODUCTION TO WEIGHT REDUCING MEALS

A portion of the weight of the obese person consists of water bound to sodium in his tissues. This excess water may be liberated and excreted during the maintenance of the low- sodium diet. In addition, the low-sodium diet tends to decrease the hydrochloric acid production in the stomach thereby decreasing hunger. The low-sodium diets for reducing which follow will be found to be of inestimable help in the program of weight reduction.

MENUS 21-30
WEIGHT REDUCING MEALS
400 - 500 Milligrams of Sodium Below 1200 Calories

MENU 21
BREAKFAST

	Milligrams Sodium	Calories
4 oz. Orange Juice (½ cup)	2.0	44
¼ cup Oatmeal (1 oz.)	9.5	115
½ cup Milk	58.0	76
Coffee (no sugar or cream)		8
1 slice Low Sodium Bread (see Menu 1)	3.5	97
	73.0	340

LUNCH

	Milligrams Sodium	Calories
Scrambled Egg and Mushrooms (see Menu 1)	81.1	130
Salad: ½ Grapefruit, 1 oz. Lettuce	4.2	15
Cherry and Banana Gelatin	47.6	123

Coffee (no sugar or cream)		8
	132.9	276

DINNER

	Milligrams Sodium	Calories
½ lb. Broiled Liver	195.2	328
4 oz. Mashed Yellow Turnips	5.6	56
Eggplant Mexican*	23.2	40
Salad: 2 oz. lettuce and 1 medium tomato	10.0	22
Vinegar Dressing—4 t.	3.0	19
Baked Apple with	2.4	40
1 t. Sugar and Cinnamon		19
Coffee	4.8	33
	244.2	557
Total for the day	450.1	1173

----

* Asterisks denote dishes for which recipes are given.

RECIPES FOR MENU 21
CHERRY AND BANANA GELATIN (Enough for 2 servings)

	Milligrams Sodium	Calories
1 pkge. cherry gelatin (1 oz.)	94.2	120
2/3 cup water		
1/3 cup sliced bananas (2 oz.)	0.4	26
1/3 cup pitted canned black cherries (2½ oz.)	0.5	100
	95.1	246
Portion for one	47.6	123

Dissolve gelatin and water as directed. Chill until syrupy. Beat until frothy. Fold in fruit and chill.

EGGPLANT MEXICAN

	Milligrams Sodium	Calories
4 oz. eggplant	2.8	16
½ cup tomatoes (4 oz.)	20.4	24
½ t. minced onion		
1/6 t. chili powder		
Pepper and bit of garlic		
	23.2	40

Pare and cut eggplant into cubes. Add remaining ingredients. Simmer 1 hour or until eggplant is tender.

MENU 22
BREAKFAST

	Milligrams Sodium	Calories
1 Orange, sliced	2.4	32
1 T. Rice (cooked) with	1.2	68
½ cup Hot Milk	58.0	76
1 slice Low Sodium Bread (see Menu 1)	3.5	97
1 t. Butter (unsalted)	0.2	38
Coffee (without cream or sugar)		8
	65.3	319

LUNCH

	Milligrams Sodium	Calories
1 Fried Egg and Mashed Potatoes (Menu 2)	72.8	249
1 cup Fruit Salad, canned (4 oz.)	10.0	80
Coffee (without cream or sugar)		8
	82.8	337

DINNER

	Milligrams Sodium	Calories

	Milligrams Sodium	Calories
½ lb. Broiled Shoulder Lamb Chops, lean only (weighed with fat and bone)	136.0	288
4 oz. Boiled Peas		56
Boiled Parsley Potato	4.0	92
3 oz. Celery Hearts (about 2)	116.7	9
4 t. Vinegar Dressing (Menu 21)	3.0	19
Canned Pears, 2 halves (4 oz.)	9.2	72
Coffee —2 t. milk and 1 t. sugar	4.8	33
	273.7	569
Total for the day	421.8	1225

MENU 23
BREAKFAST

	Milligrams Sodium	Calories
½ Grapefruit, sliced (4 oz.)	0.8	12
1 Shredded Wheat Biscuit (1 oz.)	4.7	103
½ Bananas (2½ oz.) with	0.5	33
½ cup Milk.	58.0	76
1 slice Low Sodium Bread (see Menu I)	3.5	97
Coffee (without cream or sugar)		8
	67.5	329

LUNCH

	Milligrams Sodium	Calories
Spanish Omelet (Menu 3)	93.0	136
1 slice Low Sodium Bread (see Menu I)	3.5	97
1 cup canned Pineapple (5 oz.)	1.4	90
Coffee (without cream or sugar)		8
	97.9	331

DINNER

	Milligrams Sodium	Calories

	Milligrams Sodium	Calories
Cod—Sweet and Sour (Menu 19)	213.5	171
Baked Potato	8.2	96
Diced Carrots with Minted Peas (Menu 3)	28.9	65
Hearts of Lettuce (2 oz.)	6.8	6
4 t. Vinegar Dressing (Menu 21)	3.0	19
Pineapple and Cocoanut (Menu 3)	3.4	123
	263.8	480
Total for the day	429.2	1140

MENU 24
BREAKFAST

	Milligrams Sodium	Calories
8 oz. Orange Juice	4.0	88
1 cup Puffed Rice (½ oz.)	0.1	60
½ cup Milk	58.0	76
Coffee-2 t milk and 1 t. sugar	4.8	33
	66.9	257

LUNCH

	Milligrams Sodium	Calories
Mushroom Omelet (see Menu 4)	73.8	127
2 oz. Lettuce and ½ Tomato	8.0	14
1 slice Low Sodium Bread (see Menu 1)	3.5	97
1 t. Butter	0.2	38
Coffee (without cream or sugar)		8
	85.5	284

DINNER

	Milligrams Sodium	Calories
½ Grapefruit with 1 t. Honey	2.3	39
Meat Loaf (Menu 13)	255.1	297
1 Boiled Parsley Potato	4.0	92

Endive Salad (¼ small head)	2.6	1
4 t. Vinegar Dressing (see Menu 21)	3.0	19
Apple Sauce Supreme (see Menu 4)	30.7	86
Coffee - 2 t milk and 1 t. sugar	4.8	33
	302.5	567
Total for the day	454.9	1108

MENU 25
BREAKFAST

	Milligrams Sodium	Calories
4 oz. Strawberries, with	1.6	28
1 t. Sugar		19
1 can Puffed Wheat (½ oz.)	0.4	55
½ Banana, cut into Cereal	0.4	26
½ cup Milk	58.0	76
Coffee (without cream or sugar)		8
	60.4	212

LUNCH

	Milligrams Sodium	Calories
Asparagus Omelet (Menu 16)	68.1	87
1 Roll (Menu 5)	8.0	77
Salad: ½ orange, 2 oz. lettuce	8.0	22
Coffee — 2 t. milk and 1 t. sugar	4.8	33
	88.9	219

DINNER

	Milligrams Sodium	Calories
8 oz. Breaded Veal Cutlet (Menu 5)	240.8	488
1 Baked Potato	8.0	96
4 oz. Brussel Sprouts (Menu 5)		69
Salad: ½ cucumber, 2 oz. lettuce,	9.1	22

½ tomato, ¼ green pepper

4 oz. Fruit Salad (canned)	8.8	80
Coffee (without cream or sugar)	10.0	8
	276.7	763
Total for the day	426.0	1194

MENU 26
BREAKFAST

	Milligrams Sodium	Calories
4 0z. Apricot Nectar (½ cup)	2.0	68
¼ cup Instant Ralston (1 oz.) with	0.2	110
½ cup Milk	58.0	76
Coffee — 2 t. milk and 1 t. sugar	4.8	33
	65.0	287

LUNCH

	Milligrams Sodium	Calories
Spicy Creamed Egg (Menu VI)	106.5	225
1 Boiled Mashed Potato	4.0	92
Salad: ½ apple, ½ grapefruit (sliced) on 1 leaf lettuce		8
Coffee (without Sugar or Cream)		8
	115.9	360

DINNER

	Milligrams Sodium	Calories
Braised Veal Chop, shoulder (Menu XVII)	244.9	315
Baked Potato	8.0	96
1 t. Butter	0.2	38
2 oz. Hearts of Lettuce	6.8	6
4 t. Vinegar Dressing (Menu XXI)	3.0	19
Apple Sauce, ½ cup (4½ oz.)	0.4	45

	Milligrams Sodium	Calories
Coffee — 2 t. milk and 1 t. sugar	4.8	33
	268.1	552
Total for the day	449.0	1199

MENU 27
BREAKFAST

	Milligrams Sodium	Calories
1 Orange, sliced	2.4	32
1 cup Puffed Rice (½ oz.) with	0.1	60
2 oz. Blueberries with	0.2	30
½ cup Milk	58.0	76
1 slice Low Sodium Bread (see Menu I)	3.5	97
Coffee (without cream or sugar)		8
	64,2	303

LUNCH

	Milligrams Sodium	Calories
Spring Salad (see Menu IX)	204.3	226
1 slice Low Sodium Bread (see Menu I)	3.5	97
½ Cantaloupe (3⅓ oz.)	12.6	23
Coffee — 2 t. milk and 1 t. sugar	4.8	33
	225.2	379

DINNER

	Milligrams Sodium	Calories
½ lb. Pan-Browned Pork Chops (see Menu VII)	70.6	304
with Sauce Creole (make 2 portions, one for next day's lunch for Spaghetti)	5.0	20
1 Baked Sweet Potato	20.4	92
2½ oz. Candied Carrots (see Menu VII)	68.1	62

	Milligrams Sodium	Calories
½ oz. Endive Salad (¼ head) with	2.6	1
4 t. Vinegar Dressing (see Menu XXI)	3.0	19
Coffee (without cream or sugar)		8
	169.7	506
Total for the day	459.1	1188

MENU 28
BREAKFAST

	Milligrams Sodium	Calories
4 oz. Grapefruit Juice, unsweetened	0.4	40
2 t Farina (2/3 oz.). (Do not use the quick cooking type)	0.1	67
½ cup Milk	58.0	76
Coffee-2 t milk and 1 t. sugar	4.8	33
	61.5	202

LUNCH

	Milligrams Sodium	Calories
Scrambled Egg—1 egg (use 1 t. butter for frying)	67.2	115
2 oz. Spaghetti with	4.4	64
Creole Sauce made for Pork Chops on Menu XXVII	5.0	20
Salad: ½ tomato and 1 oz. lettuce	5.0	11
Coffee (without cream or sugar)		8
	81.6	218

DINNER

	Milligrams Sodium	Calories
Baked Chicken, ½ lb. (see Menu XIV)	216.7	509
1 Mashed Potato	4.0	92

	Milligrams Sodium	Calories
4 oz. Boiled Cabbage	25.6	28
Salad: 2 oz. lettuce and ½ sliced orange	8.0	22
Cherry and Banana Gelatin (see Menu XXI)	47.6	123
Coffee (without cream or sugar)		8
	301.9	782
Total for the day	445.0	1202

MENU 29
BREAKFAST

	Milligrams Sodium	Calories
½ Grapefruit	0.8	12
¼ cup Maltex Cereal	1.1	110
½ cup Milk	58.0	76
Coffee (without cream or sugar)		8
	59.9	206

LUNCH

	Milligrams Sodium	Calories
Strained Vegetable Soup (see Menu 9)	62.3	133
French Omelet (see Menu 9)	67.2	115
Salad: 1 oz. cucumber, 1 oz. lettuce, ½ tomato	8.7	14
4 t. Vinegar Dressing (see Menu 21)	3.0	19
1 Roll (see Menu 5)	8.0	77
Coffee (without cream or sugar)		8
	149.2	366

DINNER

	Milligrams Sodium	Calories
Baked Cod in Milk (see Menu 9)	229.7	394

	Milligrams Sodium	Calories
1 Boiled Potato	4.0	92
Eggplant Mexican (see Menu 21)	23.2	40
Salad: ½ sliced apple, ½ sliced banana, shredded lettuce leaf	5.1	56
Coffee (without cream or sugar)		8
	262.0	590
Total for the day	471.1	1162

MENU 30
BREAKFAST

	Milligrams Sodium	Calories
4 oz. Canned Pears (2 halves)	9.2	72
1 Boiled Egg	67.0	77
1 Roll (see Menu 5)	8.0	77
1 t. Butter	0.2	38
Coffee — 2 t. milk and 1 t. sugar	4.8	33
	89.2	297

LUNCH

	Milligrams Sodium	Calories
Cucumbers in Sour Cream (see Menu 10)	15.6	129
1 Roll (see Menu 5)	8.0	77
Cantaloupe Gelatin Salad (see Menu 17)	17.4	73
Coffee — 2 t. milk and 1 t. sugar	4.8	33
	45.8	312

DINNER

	Milligrams Sodium	Calories
Liver Saute	125.	270
1 Baked Potato and 1 t. Butter	8.2	134
¼ lb. Buttered Spring Beans and 1	3.8	46

t. Butter

Stuffed Celery (see Menu 15)	112.7	25
2½ oz. Ice Cream (1 gill)	71.2	145
	320.9	620
Total for the day	455.9	1229

RECIPE FOR MENU 30
LIVER SAUTE

	Milligrams Sodium	Calories
4 oz. calf's liver, dredged in flour	124.0	228
Flour		20
1/6 onion chopped	0.9	
1 peppercorn and pepper		3
½ t. butter	0.1	19
Bit of bay leaf and shredded lemon peel		
	125.0	270

Wash liver in cold water. Rub with pepper. Dredge with flour and brown quickly in browned butter. Add onion, bay leaf, lemon peel, 2 T. water and peppercorn. Cover pot and cook slowly 20 minutes or until tender. Remove to hot platter and strain gravy over the meat. Garnish with chopped parsley.

MENUS 31-40

WEIGHT REDUCING MENUS
Less than 350 Milligrams of Sodium Calories below 1200

MENU 31
BREAKFAST

Milligrams   Calories

	Sodium	
4 oz. Orange Juice (½ cup)	2.0	44
¼ cup Oatmeal (1 oz.)	9.5	115
½ cup Milk	58.0	76
1 slice Low Sodium Bread (see Menu 1)	3.5	97
Coffee (without cream or sugar)		8
	73.0	340

LUNCH

	Milligrams Sodium	Calories
Scrambled Eggs and Mushrooms (see Menu 1)	81.1	130
Salad: ½ grapefruit, 1 oz. lettuce	4.2	15
3 canned Prunes (3⅓ oz.)	2.8	100
Coffee (without cream or sugar)		8
	88.1	253

DINNER

	Milligrams Sodium	Calories
6 oz. Broiled Liver	146.4	246
4 oz. fresh Boiled Peas		56
4 oz. Mashed Yellow Turnips	5.6	56
Salad: 2 oz. lettuce and 1 medium tomato	10.0	22
4 t. Vinegar Dressing (see Menu 21)	3.0	19
Baked Apple with	2.4	40
1 t. Sugar and Cinnamon		19
Coffee — 2 t. milk and 1 t. sugar	4.8	33
	172.2	491
Total for the day	333.3	1084

MENU 32
BREAKFAST

	Milligrams Sodium	Calories
1 Orange, sliced	2.4	32
1 T. Rice (cooked) with	1.2	68
½ cup Milk, hot	58.0	76
1 slice Low Sodium Bread (see Menu 1)	3.5	97
1 t. Butter (unsalted)	0.2	38
Coffee (without cream or sugar)		8
	65.3	319

LUNCH

	Milligrams Sodium	Calories
1 Fried Egg and Mashed Potatoes (see Menu 2)	72.8	249
1 cup Fruit Salad, canned (4 oz.)	10.0	80
Coffee (without cream or sugar)		8
	82.8	337

DINNER

	Milligrams Sodium	Calories
½ lb. Broiled Shoulder Lamb Chops, lean only (weighed with fat and bone)	136.0	288
4 oz. Boiled Peas		56
1 Boiled Parsley Potato	4.0	92
Salad: 1 oz. cucumber, ½ tomato and 1 oz. lettuce	8.7	14
4 t. Vinegar Dressing (see Menu 21)	3.0	19
2 halves Canned Pears (4 oz.)	9.2	72
	160.9	541
Total for the day	309.0	1197

86

MENU 33
BREAKFAST

	Milligrams Sodium	Calories
½ Grapefruit, sliced (4 oz.)	0.8	12
1 Shredded Wheat Biscuit (1 oz.) with	4.7	103
½ Banana (2½ oz.) with	0.5	33
½ cup Milk	58.0	76
1 slice Low Sodium Bread (see Menu 1)	3.5	97
Coffee (without cream or sugar)		8
	67.5	329

LUNCH

	Milligrams Sodium	Calories
Spanish Omelet (see Menu 3)	93.0	136
1 slice Low Sodium Bread (see Menu 1)	3.5	97
1 cup Canned Pineapple (5 oz.)	1.4	90
Coffee — 2 t. milk and 1 t. sugar	4.8	33
	102.7	356

DINNER

	Milligrams Sodium	Calories
Broiled Flounder (see Menu 15)	118.0	159
Baked Potato	8.2	96
Diced Carrots with Minted Peas (see Menu 3)	28.9	65
Hearts of Lettuce (2 oz.)	6.8	6
4 t. Vinegar Dressing (see Menu 21)	3.0	19
Pineapple and Cocoanut (see Menu 3)	3.4	123
	168.	468

Total for the day	338.5	1153

MENU 34
BREAKFAST

	Milligrams Sodium	Calories
8 oz. Orange Juice	4.0	88
1 cup Puffed Rice (½ oz.)	0.1	60
½ cup Milk	58.0	76
Coffee — 2 t. milk and 1 t. sugar	4.8	33
	66.9	257

LUNCH

	Milligrams Sodium	Calories
Mushroom Omelet (see Menu 4)	73.8	127
2 oz. Lettuce and ½ Tomato	8.4	14
1 slice Low Sodium Bread (see Menu 1)	3.5	97
1 t. Butter	0.2	38
Coffee (without cream or sugar)		8
	85.9	284

DINNER

	Milligrams Sodium	Calories
½ Grapefruit with 1 t. Honey	2.3	39
Beef Stew (2/3 recipe for today, 1/3 for tomorrow's lunch) (see Menu 4)	151.4	386
1 slice Low Sodium Bread (see Menu 1)	3.5	97
Endive Salad (¼ small head)	2.6	1
4 t. Vinegar Dressing (see Menu 21)	3.0	19

	Milligrams Sodium	Calories
4 T. Canned Pineapple (1¼ oz.)	0.3	22
Coffee (without cream or sugar)		8
	163.1	572
Total for the day	315.9	1113

MENU 35
BREAKFAST

	Milligrams Sodium	Calories
4 oz. Strawberries with	1.6	28
1 t. Sugar		17
1 cup Puffed Wheat (½ oz.)	0.4	55
½ Banana cut into Cereal	0.4	26
½ cup Milk	58.0	76
Coffee (without cream or sugar)		8
	60.4	210

LUNCH

	Milligrams Sodium	Calories
Beef Stew, left from yesterday's meal (see Menu 4)	76.0	193
1 Roll (see Menu 5)	8.0	77
Salad: ½ orange, 2 oz. lettuce	8.0	22
Coffee — 2 t. milk and 1 t. sugar	4.8	33
	96.8	325

DINNER

	Milligrams Sodium	Calories
Macaroni with Liver (see Menu 12)	79.6	231
4 oz. String Beans Boiled with	3.6	8
1 t. Butter		38
3 oz. Yellow Turnip, Boiled	4.2	42
Orange and Raisin Slaw (see Menu 17)	20.2	56

	Milligrams Sodium	Calories
2½ OZ. Ice Cream (1 gill)	71.2	145
Coffee — 2 t. milk and 1 t. sugar	4.8	33
	183.6	553
Total for the day	340.8	1088

MENU 36
BREAKFAST

	Milligrams Sodium	Calories
4 oz. Strawberries with	1.6	28
1 t. Sugar		17
1 cup Puffed Wheat (½ oz.)	0.4	55
½ Banana cut into Cereal	0.4	26
½ cup Milk	58.0	76
Coffee (without cream or sugar)		8
	60.4	210

LUNCH

	Milligrams Sodium	Calories
Beef Stew, left from yesterday's meal (see Menu 4)	76.0	193
1 Roll (see Menu 5)	8.0	77
Salad: ½ orange, 2 oz. lettuce	8.0	22
Coffee — 2 t. milk and 1 t. sugar	4.8	33
	96.8	325

DINNER

	Milligrams Sodium	Calories
Macaroni with Liver (see Menu 12)	79.6	231
4 oz. String Beans Boiled with	3.6	8
1 t. Butter		38
3 oz. Yellow Turnip, Boiled	4.2	42
Orange and Raisin Slaw (see Menu 17)	20.2	56
2½ OZ. Ice Cream (1 gill)	71.2	145
Coffee — 2 t. milk and 1 t. sugar	4.8	33

	183.6	553
Total for the day	340.8	1088

MENU 37
BREAKFAST

	Milligrams Sodium	Calories
1 Orange, sliced	2.4	32
1 cup Puffed Rice (½ oz.) with	0.1	60
2 oz. Blueberries (6 T.) with	0.2	30
½ cup Milk	58.0	76
1 slice Low Sodium Bread (see Menu 1)	3.5	97
Coffee (without cream or sugar)		8
	64.2	303

LUNCH

	Milligrams Sodium	Calories
Curried Egg and Mushrooms (see Menu 7)	78.8	242
1 slice Low Sodium Bread (see Menu 1)	3.5	97
Vegetable Salad: ½ tomato, 1 oz. green pepper, 1 oz. cucumber, 1 oz. lettuce	8.8	22
Coffee (without cream or sugar)		8
	91.1	369

DINNER

	Milligrams Sodium	Calories
½ lb. Pan-Browned Pork Chops (see Menu 7) with	70.6	304
Sauce Creole (make 2 portions, one for next day's lunch for Spaghetti)	5.0	20
1 Baked Sweet Potato	20.4	92

	Milligrams Sodium	Calories
2½ oz. Candied Carrots (see Menu 7)	68.1	62
½ oz. Endive Salad (¼ small head) with	2.6	1
4 t. Vinegar Dressing (see Menu 21)	3.0	19
Coffee (without cream or sugar)		8
	169.7	506
Total for the day	325.0	1178

MENU 38
BREAKFAST

	Milligrams Sodium	Calories
4 oz. Grapefruit Juice (unsweetened)	0.4	40
2 T. Farina (2/3 oz.—do not use the quick cooking type) with	0.1	67
½ cup Milk	58.0	76
Coffee — 2 t. milk and 1 t. sugar	4.8	33
	63.3	216

LUNCH

	Milligrams Sodium	Calories
1 Scrambled Egg in 1 t. Butter	67.2	115
2 oz. Spaghetti with	4.4	64
Creole Sauce (made for Pork Chops on Menu 37)	5.0	20
Salad: ½ tomato and 1 oz. lettuce	5.0	11
Coffee — 2 t. milk and 1 t. sugar	4.8	33
	86.4	243

DINNER

	Milligrams Sodium	Calories
6 oz. Grilled Calf's Liver	188.4	342

	Milligrams Sodium	Calories
1 Mashed Potato	4.0	92
2½ oz. Boiled Asparagus (6 spears)	1.2	12
Salad: 1 oz. cabbage and 1 oz. pineapple on lettuce	6.9	20
Spicy Baked Apple (see Menu 8)	2.1	152
Coffee — 2 t. milk and 1 t. sugar	4.8	33
	207.4	651
Total for the day	357.1	1110

MENU 39
BREAKFAST

	Milligrams Sodium	Calories
½ Grapefruit	0.8	12
¼ cup Maltex Cereal	1.0	110
½ cup Milk	58.0	76
Coffee — 2 t. milk and 1 t. sugar	4.8	33
	64.6	231

LUNCH

	Milligrams Sodium	Calories
Strained Vegetable Soup (see Menu 9)	62.3	133
French Omelet (see Menu 9)	67.2	115
Salad: 1 oz. cucumber, 1 oz. lettuce, ½ tomato	8.7	14
4 t. Vinegar Dressing (see Menu 21)	3.0	19
1 Roll (see Menu 5)	8.0	77
Coffee (without cream or sugar)		8
	149.2	366

DINNER

	Milligrams Sodium	Calories

	Milligrams Sodium	Calories
Broiled Flounder (see Menu 15)	118.0	159
1 Boiled Potato	4.0	92
Fried Eggplant (see Menu 9)	5.8	138
Salad: ½ sliced apple, ½ sliced banana, shredded lettuce leaf	5.1	56
Pineapple and Cocoanut (see Menu 3)	3.4	123
Coffee (without cream or sugar)		8
	136.3	576
Total for the day	350.1	1173

MENU 40
BREAKFAST

	Milligrams Sodium	Calories
4 oz. Canned Pears (2 halves)	9.2	72
1 Boiled Egg	67.0	77
1 Roll (see Menu 5)	8.0	77
1 t. Butter	0.2	38
Coffee —2 t. milk and 1 t. sugar	4.8	33
	89.2	297

LUNCH

	Milligrams Sodium	Calories
Cucumbers in Sour Cream (see Menu 10)	15.6	129
1 Roll (see Menu 5)	8.0	77
Cantaloupe Gelatin Salad (see Menu 17)	17.4	73
Coffee (without cream or sugar)		8
	41.0	287

DINNER

	Milligrams Sodium	Calories
Liver Saute (see Menu 30)	125.0	270

1 Baked Potato with	8.0	96
1 t. Butter	0.2	38
¼ lb. String Beans	3.6	8
Salad: ½ apple, ½ Grapefruit, slices on Lettuce leaf	5.4	35
2¼ oz. Ice Cream (1 gill)	71.2	145
	213.4	592
Total for the day	343.6	1176

MENUS 41-50

Below 350 Milligrams of Sodium 1800 - 2200 Calories

MENU 41
BREAKFAST

	Milligrams Sodium	Calories
8 oz. Orange Juice (1 cup)	4.0	88
¼ cup Oatmeal (1 oz.)	9.5	115
½ cup Milk	58.0	76
Coffee — 2 t. cream and 1 t. sugar	3.8	65
1 slice Low Sodium Bread (see Menu 1)	3.5	97
½ T. Marmalade	2.6	37
	81.4	478

LUNCH

	Milligrams Sodium	Calories
Scrambled Eggs and Mushrooms (see Menu 1)	81.1	130
Salad: ½ grapefruit, 1 oz. lettuce	4.2	15
3 Canned Prunes (3⅓ oz.)	2.8	100
1 slice Low Sodium Bread (see Menu 1)	3.5	97

	Milligrams Sodium	Calories
1 t. Butter (unsalted)	0.2	38
Coffee — 2 t. cream and 1 t. sugar	3.8	65
	95.6	445

DINNER

	Milligrams Sodium	Calories
6 oz. Broiled Liver	146.4	246
4 oz. Boiled Peas		56
1 Boiled Potato with	4.0	92
1 t. Butter (unsalted)	0.2	38
Salad: ½ banana sliced, ½ apple sliced, 1 leaf lettuce	5.1	56
1 T. French Dressing (see Menu 3)		88
Apple Pie—1/8 slice of Pie (see Menu 4)	2.9	388
Coffee — 2 t. cream and 1 t. sugar	3.8	65
	162.4	1029
Total for the day	339.4	1952

MENU 42
BREAKFAST

	Milligrams Sodium	Calories
4 oz. Orange Juice and ½ Banana sliced	2.5	77
1 T. Rice (cooked)	1.2	68
½ cup Milk, hot	58.0	76
1 t. Sugar and Cinamon may be added to Milk		19
1 slice Low Sodium Bread (see Menu 1)	3.5	97
2 t. Jelly	4.8	49

| Coffee — 2 t. cream and 1 t. sugar | 3.8 | 65 |
| | 73.8 | 451 |

LUNCH

	Milligrams Sodium	Calories
1 Fried Egg and Mashed Potato (see Menu 2)	72.8	249
4 oz. Boiled Fresh Asparagus with	2.0	20
I T. Melted Butter	0.7	113
1 slice Low Sodium Bread (see Menu 1)	3.5	97
1 cup Fruit Salad, canned (4 oz.)	10.0	80
Coffee — 2 t. cream and 1 t. sugar	3.8	65
	92.8	624

DINNER

	Milligrams Sodium	Calories
½ Grapefruit	0.8	12
½ lb. Broiled Shoulder Lamb Chops, lean only (weighed with fat and bone)	136.0	288
4 oz. Boiled Peas		56
1 Boiled Parsley Potato	4.0	92
Salad: 1 oz. cucumber, ½ tomato and 1 oz. lettuce	8.7	14
4 t. Vinegar Dressing (see Menu 1)	3.0	63
Cantaloupe Gelatin Salad with French Dressing for Fruit Salad (see Menu 17)	18.4	207
Coffee — 2 t. cream and 1 t. sugar	3.8	65
	174.7	797
Total for the day	341.3	1872

MENU 43
BREAKFAST

	Milligrams Sodium	Calories
Mix 4 oz. Orange and 4 oz. of Grapefruit Juice	2.4	84
1 Shredded Wheat Biscuit (1 oz.) with	4.7	103
½ Banana (2½ oz.) with	0.5	33
½ cup Milk	58.0	76
1 slice Low Sodium Bread (see Menu 1)	3.5	97
1 t. Butter (unsalted)	0.2	38
Coffee — 2 t. cream and 1 t. sugar	3.8	65
	73.1	496

LUNCH

	Milligrams Sodium	Calories
Spanish Omelet (see Menu 3)	93.0	136
1 slice Low Sodium Bread (see Menu 1)	3.5	97
1 t. Butter	0.2	38
Nut and Apple Tapioca (see Menu 3)	8.5	409
Coffee — 2 t. cream and 1 t. sugar	3.8	65
	109.0	745

DINNER

	Milligrams Sodium	Calories
Broiled Flounder (see Menu 15)	118.0	159
Baked Potato with 1 t. Butter	8.2	134
Diced Carrots with Minted Peas (see Menu 3)	28.9	65
Hearts of Lettuce (2 oz.)	6.8	6

	Milligrams Sodium	Calories
1 T. French Dressing (see Menu 3)		88
Pineapple and Cocoanut (see Menu 3)	3.4	123
Coffee — 2 t. cream and 1 t. sugar	3.8	65
	169.1	640
Total for the day	351.2	1881

MENU 44
BREAKFAST

	Milligrams Sodium	Calories
8 oz. Orange Juice	4.0	88
1 cup Puffed Rice (½ oz.)	0.1	60
½ cup Milk	58.0	76
1 slice Low Sodium Bread (see Menu 1)	3.5	97
1 t. Butter	0.2	38
Coffee — 2 t. cream and 1 t. sugar	3.8	65
	69.6	424

LUNCH

	Milligrams Sodium	Calories
Mushroom Omelet (see Menu 4)	73.8	127
2 oz. Lettuce and ½ Tomato	8.4	14
1 t. French Dressing (see Menu 3)		88
1 slice Low Sodium Bread (see Menu 1)	3.5	97
1 t. Butter	0.2	38
Coffee — 2 t. cream and 1 t. sugar	3.8	65
	89.7	429

DINNER

	Milligrams	Calories

	Sodium	
½ Grapefruit with 1 t. Honey	2.3	39
Beef Stew (2/3 of recipe for today, for tomorrow's lunch—see Menu 4)	151.4	386
1 slice Low Sodium Bread (see Menu 1)	3.5	97
Endive Salad (¼ small head)	2.6	1
1 T. French Dressing (see Menu 3)		88
Nut and Apple Tapioca (see Menu 3)	8.5	409
Coffee — 2 t. cream and 1 t. sugar	3.8	65
	172.1	1085
Total for the day	331.4	1938

MENU 45
BREAKFAST

	Milligrams Sodium	Calories
8 oz. Pineapple Juice	0.8	188
1 cup Puffed Wheat (½ oz.)	0.4	55
1/9 Banana cut into Cereal	0.4	26
½ cup Milk	58.0	76
1 Roll (see Menu 5)	8.0	77
1 t. Butter	0.2	38
Coffee — 2 t. cream and 1 t. sugar	3.8	65
	71.6	481

LUNCH

	Milligrams Sodium	Calories
Beef Stew left over from yesterday's dinner on Menu 44	76.0	193
1 Hot Roll	8.0	77
1 t. Butter	0.2	38
Salad: ½ orange, 2 oz. lettuce	8.0	22

	Milligrams Sodium	Calories
1 T. French Dressing (see Menu 3)		88
4 oz. Canned Peaches (2 halves)	6.8	76
Coffee-2 t. cream and 1 t. sugar	3.8	65
	102.8	559

DINNER

	Milligrams Sodium	Calories
Macaroni with Liver (see Menu 12)	79.6	231
4 oz. Pan-Fried Potatoes (see Menu 5)	8.0	316
4 oz. Brussels Sprouts (see Menu 5)	9.1	69
Salad: ½ cucumber, 2 oz. lettuce, ½ tomato, ¼ green pepper	8.8	22
Custard Cake Pudding (see Menu 5)	34.5	317
Coffee — 2 t. cream and 1 t. sugar	3.8	65
	143.8	1020
Total for the day	318.2	2060

MENU 46
BREAKFAST

	Milligrams Sodium	Calories
8 oz. Apricot Nectar	4.0	136
¼ cup Instant Ralston	0.2	110
½ cup Milk with	58.0	76
1 T. Raisins	5.0	23
1 slice Low Sodium Bread (see Menu 1)	3.5	97
1 t. Butter	0.2	38
Coffee - 2 t cream and 1 t. sugar	3.8	65
	74.7	545

LUNCH

	Milligrams Sodium	Calories
Spicy Creamed Egg (see Menu 6)	106.5	225
1 Boiled Mashed Potato	4.0	92
Salad: ½ apple sliced, ½ grapefruit sliced on 1 leaf lettuce	5.4	35
Peach Cocketail (see Menu 6)	6.0	99
Coffee — 2 t. cream and 1 t. sugar	3.8	65
	125.7	516

DINNER

	Milligrams Sodium	Calories
6 oz. Broiled Sirloin Steak	117.6	300
1 Baked Potato	8.0	96
1 t. Butter	0.2	38
4 oz. Boiled Peas	4.0	56
2 oz. Hearts of Lettuce	6.8	6
1 T. French Dressing (see Menu 3)		88
Banana and Grape Gelatin (see Menu 18)	2.4	106
Coffee - 2 t cream and 1 t. sugar	3.8	65
	142.8	755
Total for the day	343.2	1816

MENU 47
BREAKFAST

	Milligrams Sodium	Calories
1 Orange, sliced	2.4	32
1 cup Puffed Rice	0.1	60
2 oz. Blueberries, with	0.2	30
½ cup Milk	58.0	76
1 slice Low Sodium Bread, toasted (see Menu 1)	3.5	97
1 t. Butter	0.2	38

1 T. Marmalade	5.2	74
Coffee — 2 t. cream and 1 t. sugar	3.8	65
	73.4	472

LUNCH

	Milligrams Sodium	Calories
Curried Egg and Mushrooms (see Menu 7)	78.8	242
1 slice Low Sodium Bread	3.5	97
1 t. Butter	0.2	38
Vegetable Salad: ½ tomato, 1 oz. lettuce, 1 oz. green pepper, 1 oz. cucumber	8.8	22
Coffee — 2 t. cream and 1 t. sugar	3.8	65
3 Seed Cookies (see Menu 7)	12.0	255
	107.1	719

DINNER

	Milligrams Sodium	Calories
½ lb. Pan-Broiled Pork Chops (see Menu 7) with	70.6	304
Sauce Creole (make 2 portions, one for next day's lunch for Spaghetti)	5.0	20
1 Baked Potato with 1 t. Butter	8.2	134
2½ oz. Candied Carrots (see Menu 7)	68.1	6
½ oz. Endive Salad (¼ small head) with	2.6	1
1 T. French Dressing (see Menu 3)		88
Coffee — 2 t. cream and 1 t. sugar	3.8	65
2 Seed Cookies (see Menu 7)	8.0	170
	166.3	844

Total for the day	346.8	2035

MENU 48
BREAKFAST

	Milligrams Sodium	Calories
4 oz. Grapefruit Juice (unsweetened)	0.4	40
2 T. Farina (2/3 oz.—do not use quick-cooking type)	0.1	67
½ cup Milk	58.0	76
1 slice Cinnamon Toast (see Menu 1)	3.5	97
1 t. Butter	0.2	38
Coffee — 2 t. cream and 1 t. sugar	3.8	65
	66.0	383

LUNCH

	Milligrams Sodium	Calories
1 Scrambled Egg in 1 t. Butter	67.2	115
2 oz. Spaghetti with	4.4	64
Creole Sauce (made for Pork Chops on previous day's dinner)	5.0	20
Coffee — 2 t. cream and 1 t. sugar	3.8	65
2 Sugar Cookies (see Menu 8)	0.6	136
	81.0	400

DINNER

	Milligrams Sodium	Calories
6 oz. Grilled Calf's Liver	188.4	342
1 Boiled Mashed Potato with	4.0	92
1 t. Butter	0.2	38
4 oz. Green Peas with 1 t. Butter	0.6	94
Salad: ½ apple, ½ sliced	5.4	35

grapefruit on 1 oz. Lettuce

French Dressing for Fruit Salad (see Menu 17)	1.0	134
Spicy Baked Apple (see Menu 8)	2.1	152
Coffee — 2 t. cream and 1 t. sugar	3.8	65
2 Sugar Cookies (see Menu 8)	0.6	136
	206.1	1088
Total for the day	353.1	1871

MENU 49
BREAKFAST

	Milligrams Sodium	Calories
½ Grapefruit	0.8	12
¼ cup Maltex Wheat Cereal (1 oz.)	1.0	110
2 canned Prunes (2 oz.)	1.7	60
½ cup Milk	58.0	76
1 Hot Roll (see Menu 5)	8.0	77
1 t. Butter	0.2	38
Coffee — 2 t. cream and 1 t. sugar	3.8	65
	73.5	438

LUNCH

	Milligrams Sodium	Calories
French Omelet (see Menu 9)	67.2	115
1 Boiled Potato with	4.0	92
1 t. Butter	0.2	38
Salad: 1 oz. cucumber, 1 oz. lettuce, ½ tomato	8.7	14
1 T. French Dressing (see Menu 3)		88
Pineapple and Cocoanut (see	3.4	123

Menu 3)

	Milligrams Sodium	Calories
Coffee — 2 t. cream and 1 t. sugar	3.8	65
	87.3	535

DINNER

	Milligrams Sodium	Calories
Broiled Flounder (see Menu 15)	118.0	159
1 Boiled Potato	4.0	92
Fried Eggplant (see Menu 9)	5.8	138
Salad: ½ sliced apple, ½ sliced banana, 1 shredded lettuce leaf	5.1	56
French Dressing for Fruit Salad (see Menu 17)	1.0	134
Custard Cake Pudding (see Menu 5)	34.5	317
Coffee — 2 t. cream and 1 t. sugar	3.8	65
	172.2	961
Total for the day	333.0	1934

MENU 50
BREAKFAST

	Milligrams Sodium	Calories
4 oz. canned Pears (2 halves)	9.2	72
¼ cup Wheatena (1 oz.)	0.2	110
½ cup Milk (hot)	58.0	76
Spiced with 1 t. Sugar and bit of Cinnamon		18
1 Roll (see Menu 5)	8.0	77
2 t. Butter	0.4	76
Coffee — 2 t. cream and 1 t. sugar	3.8	65
	79.6	494

LUNCH

	Milligrams Sodium	Calories
Cucumber in Sour Cream (see Menu 10)	15.6	129
1 Roll (see Menu 5)	8.0	77
1 t. Butter	0.2	38
Cantaloupe Gelatin Salad (see Menu 17)	17.4	73
French Dressing for Fruit Salad (see Menu 17)	1.0	134
Coffee — 2 t. cream and 1 t. sugar	3.8	65
	46.0	516

DINNER

	Milligrams Sodium	Calories
4 oz. Liver Saute (see Menu 30)	125	270
1 Baked Potato with	8.0	96
1 t. Butter	0.2	38
¼ lb. String Beans with	3.6	8
1 t. Butter	0.2	38
Salad: ½ Apple, ½ grapefruit slices on 1 lettuce leaf	5.4	35
French Dressing for Fruit Salad (see Menu 17)	1.0	134
Sweet Pilau (see Men 15)	25.8	501
Coffee — 2 t. cream and 1 t. sugar	3.8	65
	173.0	1185
Total for the day	298.6	2195

LOW SODIUM DIETS FOR THE PERSON WHO EATS OUT

If obliged to have lunch or dinner out, the patient is faced with rather a difficult problem. He will be obliged to limit his menu to more or less the same type of food each day. A few sample meals which may be obtained in a restaurant follow:

MENU A

	Milligrams Sodium	Calories
½ Grapefruit	0.8	12
2 Boiled Eggs	134.4	154
Salad: 2 oz. lettuce, ½ tomato	8.0	14
Dressing: Vinegar and Sugar	3.0	19
Coffee — 2 t. cream and 1 t. sugar	3.8	65
Baked Apple	2.4	59
	152.4	323

MENU B

	Milligrams Sodium	Calories
8 oz. Steak (broiled)	156.8	400
1 Baked Potato (1 t. Butter, unsalted)	8.2	134
Salad: No dressing except vinegar, sugar, and oil	11.0	33
2½ oz. Ice Cream (1 gill)	71.2	145
Coffee — 2 t. cream and 1 t. sugar	3.8	65
	251.0	777

MENU C

	Milligrams Sodium	Calories
Fruit Cup	5.0	40
4 oz. Lamb Chops, broiled	13.6	212

	Milligrams Sodium	Calories
Baked Potato (1 t. Butter, unsalted)	8.2	134
Salad: No dressing except vinegar or sugar and oil	11.0	33
Canned Pineapple	1.4	90
Coffee — 2 t. cream and 1 t. sugar	3.8	65
	133.0	574

MENU D

	Milligrams Sodium	Calories
½ lb. Broiled Liver		
1 Baked Potato		
Salad: No dressing except vinegar or sugar and oil	11.0	
1 cup Fruit Salad (may be canned)		
Coffee — 2 t. cream and 1 t. sugar		
	228.0	602

MENU E

	Milligrams Sodium	Calories
½ Grapefruit		
½ lb. Broiled Lamb Chops (shoulder)		
1 Baked Potato (1 t. Butter, unsalted)		
Salad: No dressing except vinegar, sugar or oil	11.0	
4 oz. Canned Peaches (or other fruit)		
Coffee — 2 t. cream and 1 t. sugar		
	166.6	608

The secret of eating out lies in the use of Jewish unleavened bread, called Matzoth. This is a tasty and satisfying substitute for bread. However, be sure to buy the plain Matzoth marked "Passover," which is traditionally made without salt.

Tea Matzoth, which contains slightly more sodium than the Passover Matzoth, will be found to be a very pleasant variation.

Care must be taken, however, to avoid such preparations as poppy seed Matzoths, tasty wafer Matzoths, and whole wheat Matzoths, as well as Matzoths, American Style.

THE SALT-FREE DIET FOR THE DIABETIC

One of the most frequent complications of diabetes is arteriosclerotic vascular disease. Adequate diets are available to the person with uncomplicated diabetes. The diabetic, however, who suffers from hypertension requires the special type of sodium-free diet suggested in this book. It is, of course, expected that he will not attempt self-treatment, but will consult with his physician in the selection of the diet best suited to him.

All fruits must be water packed.
No salt is to be added to any food.
Cream to be used should be 20%.
All canned foods must be salt free.

There may be slight variations between the calories listed on the Diabetic Salt-Free Diets and the ones preceding. This slight difference is due to our use of Food and Beverage Analysis by Bridges and Mattice for our authority on analysis for the Diabetic Menus.

SUMMARY OF THE MENUS AND THEIR VALUES

Menu	Carb.	Prot.	Fats	Cal.	Mg. na.
A	127.0	68.2	68.3	1436	358.3
B	128.8	66.2	78.8	1536	324.9
C	135.3	63.9	76.2	1530	262.4
D	149.7	73.7	83.7	1683	319.1

E	160.3	77.4	92.5	1823	348.8
F	147.5	75.7	85.8	1688	320.0
G	140.0	90.7	98.1	1821	423.2
H	185.3	79.7	77.2	1787	409.6
I	199.8	99.3	90.7	2051	432.1

MENU A

BREAKFAST

	Carb	Prot.	Fat	Cal.	Mg. Na.
4 oz. Canned Pears (2 halves) (Water packed)	4.9	.4	.1	25	8.8
¼ c Wheatena (1 oz.)	21.7	3.2	.8	110	.2
½ c. Milk	6.0	3.9	4.8	85	58.0
1 Slice Low Sodium Bread (Menu 1)	18.2	2.9	1.5	101	3.5
2 t. Butter			5.6	54	.4
Coffee with 1 T. Cream	2.3	.9	3.0	39	5.7
	53.1	11.3	15.8	414	76.6

LUNCH

	Carb	Prot.	Fat	Cal.	Mg. Na.
One Sliced Hard Boiled Egg on		6.7	5.2	75	67
2 oz. Lettuce	0.5	0.6	.2	6	6.8
Cucumbers in Sour Cream (Menu 10)	4.7	1.2	6.0	77	15.6
Coffee with 1 T. Cream	2.3	0.9	3.0	39	5.7
	7.5	9.4	14.4	197	95.1

DINNER

	Carb	Prot.	Fat	Cal.	Mg. Na.
8 oz. Steak, Broiled, Fat not to be eaten		33.9	6.9	205	156.8
1 Baked Potato (5 oz.)	38.1	4.6	.1	175	10

	Carb.	Prot.	Fat	Cal.	Mg. Na.
1 t. Butter			2.8	27	.2
¾ c. String Beans (2½ oz.)	5.8	1.8	.2	35	4.5
2 t. Butter			5.6	54	.2
Salad, ½ Apple, ½ Grapefruit slices on Lettuce Leaf, with	11.6	1.1	.3	55	6.0
3 Chopped Walnuts	1.8	4.8	9.8	88	.4
1 T. French Dressing (Menu 3)	.4	.4	9.3	30	2.8
3 Prunes, Water packed	6.4	.9	.1	39	5.7
Coffee with 1 T. Cream	2.3	47.5	3.0	825	186.6
	66.4	68.2	38.1	1436	358.3
Total for the day	127.0	33.9	68.3	205	156.8

MENU B

BREAKFAST

	Carb.	Prot.	Fat	Cal.	Mg. Na.
1 Orange, Sliced	8.5	.8	.2	40	2.4
1 c. Puffed Rice (½ oz.) with	13.3	.9		60	.1
2 oz. Blueberries, with	5.4	.2	.2	25	.2
½ c. Milk	6.0	3.9	4.8	85	58.0
1 t. Butter			2.8	27	.2
1 Slice Low Sodium Bread (Menu 1)	18.2	2.9	1.5	101	3.5
Coffee with 1 T. Cream	2.3	.9	3.0	39	5.7
	53.7	9.6	12.5	377	70.1

LUNCH

	Carb	Prot.	Fat	Cal.	Mg. Na.
Curried Egg and Mushroom (Menu 7)	3.1	7.9	14.0	174	78.8
1 t. Butter			2.8	27	.2
1 Slice Low Sodium Bread	18.2	2.9	1.5	101	3.5
Vegetable Salad, ½ Tomato, 1 oz. Green Pepper, 1 oz.	3.7	1.3	.3	24	8.8

	Carb	Prot.	Fat	Cal.	Mg. Na.
Cucumbers I oz. Lettuce ½ c. Pineapple (Water packed) with	7.6	2		32	1.2
6 Soft-shell Walnuts, chopped	4.7	5.8	22.2	250	.6
Coffee with 1 T. Cream	2.3	.9	3.0	39	5.7
	39.6	19.0	43.8	647	98.8

DINNER

	Carb	Prot.	Fat	Cal.	Mg. Na.
½ lb. Pan-Browned Pork Chops (Menu 7) with		32.9	8.3	215	70.6
Sauce Creole (Menu 7)	4.5	*1.0*	.4	26	5.0
1 Boiled Potato, Sprinkled with Parsley	18.0	2.2	.1	85	4.0
2½ oz. Candied Carrots (Menu 7)	9.7	.4	1.4	56	68.1
½ oz. Endive Salad	.6	2		3	2.6
I T. French Dressing (Menu 3)	.4		9.3	88	
Coffee with 1 T. Cream	2.3	.9	3.0	39	5.7
	35.5	37.6	22.5	512	156
Total for the day	128.8	66.2	78.8	1536	324.9

MENU C

BREAKFAST

	Carb	Prot.	Fat	Cal.	Mg.Na
4 oz. Canned Pears, Water packed, 2 halves	4.9	.9	.1	25	8.8
¼ c. Wheatena 1 oz	21.7	3.2	.8	110	2
½ c. Milk	6.0	3.9	4.8	85	58.0
1 Slice Low Sodium Bread (Menu 1)	18.2	2.9	1.5	101	3.5
1 t. Butter			2.8	27	.2

| Coffee with 1 T. Cream | 2.3 | .9 | 3.0 | 39 | 5.7 |
| | 53.1 | 11.3 | 13.0 | 387 | 76.4 |

LUNCH

	Carb	Prot.	Fat	Cal.	Mg.Na
Cucumbers in Sour Cream (Menu 10)	4.7	1.2	6.0	77	15.6
1 Slice Low Sodium Bread (Menu 1)	18.2	2.9	1.5	101	3.5
1 t. Butter			2.8	27	.2
Cantaloupe Gelatin Salad (Menu 17) Add 6 Soft-shelled Walnuts, Chopped fine, to the recipe	26.4	7.7	22.4	350	18.2
Coffee with 1 T. Cream	2.3	.9	3.0	39	5.7
	51.6	12.7	35.7	594	43.2

DINNER

	Carb	Prot.	Fat	Cal.	Mg.Na
4 oz. Liver, Saute (Menu 30)	9.7	34.3	18.1	351	125.0
6 Stalks Boiled Asparagus (2½ oz.)	1.2	1.8	.3	15	1.2
1 t. butter			2.8	27	2
¾ c. String Beans (2½ oz.)	5.8	1.8	.2	35	4.5
1 t. Butter			2.8	27	2
Salad, ½ Apple, ½ Grapefruit slices on Lettuce Leaf	11.6	1.1	.3	55	6.0
Coffee with 1 T. Cream	2.3	.9	3.0	39	5.7
	30.6	39.9	37.5	549	142.8
Total for the day	135.3	63.9	76.2	1530	262.4

MENU D

BREAKFAST

	Carb	Prot.	Fat	Cal.	Mg.Na
½ Small Cantaloupe (7 oz.)	10.0			40	26.6
1 c. Puffed Wheat (½ oz.)	11.3	2.3	.2	55	.4

114

	Carb	Prot.	Fat	Cal.	Mg.Na
½ Banana. cut into Cereal	13.1	0.8	.4	60	.7
4 T. Cream (20%)	2.3	1.7	12.0	124	22.8
1 Slice Low Sodium Bread (Menu 1)	18.2	2.9	1.5	101	3.5
1 t. Butter			2.8	27	.2
Coffee with 1 T. Cream	2.3	.9	3.0	39	5.7
	57.2	8.6	19.9	446	59.9

LUNCH

	Carb	Prot.	Fat	Cal.	Mg.Na
Curried Egg and Mushroom (Menu 7)	3.1	7.9	14.0	174	78.8
1 Slice Low Sodium Bread (Menu 1)	18.2	2.9	1.5	101	3.5
1 t. Butter			2.8	27	.2
Salad, ½ Tomato, 1 oz. lettuce, 1 oz. Green Pepper. 1 oz. Cucumber	3.7	1.3	.3	24	8.8
8 Cashew Nuts. Fried in coconut oil, unsalted	2.0	4.3	7.9	100	1.8
Coffee with 1 T. Cream	2.3	.9	3.0	39	5.7
	29.3	17.3	29.5	465	98.8

DINNER

	Carb	Prot.	Fat	Cal.	Mg.Na
½ lb. Broiled Shoulder Lamb Chops		35.6	8.6	225	136.0
1 Baked Potato, 5 oz. with	38.1	4.6	.1	175	10.0
1 t. Butter			2.8	27	.2
Salad, Vi Orange, 2 oz. Lettuce, 3 Walnuts	6.4	5.8	10.1	143	7.8
I T. French Dressing (Menu 3)	.4		9.3	88	
8 oz. Watermelon, 1 c. Diced	16.0	.9	.4	75	.7
Coffee with 1 T. Cream	2.3	.9	3.0	39	5.7
	63.2	47.8	34.3	772	160.4
Total for the day	149.7	73.7	83.7	1683	319.1

MENU E

BREAKFAST

	Carb	Prot.	Fat	Cal.	Mg.Na
4 or Orange Juice	11.3	.7		50	2.0
1 Shredded Wheat Biscuit with	24.5	3.3	.5	120	4.7
½ Banana (2½ or) with	13.1	.8	.4	60	.7
½ c. Milk	6.0	3.9	4.8	85	58.0
1 Slice Low Sodium Bread (Menu 1)	18.2	2.9	1.5	101	3.5
1 t. Butter			2.8	27	.2
Cofee with 1 T. Cream	2.3	.9	3.0	39	5.7
	75.4	12.5	13.0	482	74.8

LUNCH

	Carb	Prot.	Fat	Cal.	Mg.Na
Spanish Omelet (Menu 3)	9.5	9.9	5.8	130	93.0
1 Slice Low Sodium Bread (Menu 1)	8.2	2.9	1.5	101	3.5
1 t. Butter			2.8	27	.2
Coffee with 1 T. Cream	2.3	.9	3.0	39	5.7
	30.0	13.7	13.1	297	102.4

DINNER

	Carb	Prot.	Fat	Cal.	Mg.Na
Broiled Flounder (Menu 15)	1.3	32.7	4.2	178	118.0
4 or Pan-Fried Potatoes (Menu 5)	22.0	2.8	24.1	322	8.0
Diced Carrots with Minted Peas (Menu 3)	9.6	3.8	1.7	73	28.9
Hearts of Lettuce (2 ox.)	.5	.6	.2	6	6.8
1 T. French Dressing (Menu 3)	.4		9.3	88	
Pineapple and Coconut (Menu 3)	18.6	10.4	23.9	338	42
Coffee with 1 T. Cream	2.3	.9	3.0	39	5.7
	54.9	51.2	66.4	1044	171.6

116

Total for the day	160.3	77.4	923	1823	348.8

MENU F

BREAKFAST

	Carb	Prot.	Fat	Cal.	Mg.Na
8 oz. Orange Juice	22.6	1.4		100	4.0
¼ c. Oatmeal (2/3 oz.)	13.5	3.2	1.4	80	6.3
4 T. Cream (20%)	2.3	1.7	12.0	124	22.8
Coffee, with 1 T. Cream	2.3	.9	3.0	39	5.7
1 Slice Low Sodium Bread (Menu 1)	18.2	2.9	1.5	101	3.5
1 t. Butter			2.8	27	.2
	58.9	10.1	20.7	401	42.5

LUNCH

	Carb	Prot.	Fat	Cal.	Mg.Na
Scrambled Egg and Mushrooms (Menu 1) Substitute 1 T. Cream for the Milk in the recipe	.6	7.1	11.0	133	76.8
Salad, ½ Apple, ½ Banana, 1 Lettuce Leaf	19.4	1.3	.7	90	5.1
Orange Rice Custard (Menu 1) Substitute saccharine for sugar in the recipe	20.6	3.6	15.1	235	30.6
	40.6	12.0	26.8	458	112.5

DINNER

	Carb	Prot.	Fat	Cal.	Mg.Na
6 oz. Broiled Liver	4.3	35.2	9.3	232	146.4
2½ oz. Boiled Peas	8.0	4.3	.4	55	.5
1 Boiled Potato (3⅓ oz.)	18.0	2.2	.1	85	4.0
2 t. Butter			5.6	54	.4
Salad. ½ Grapefruit, 1 oz. Lettuce, 6 Chopped Walnuts	9.0	10.6	19.8	263	5.2
3 Prunes, Canned, Water-	6.4	.4	.1	30	2.8

packed

	Carb	Prot.	Fat	Cal.	Mg.Na
Coffee with 1 T. Cream	2.3	.9	3.0	40	5.7
	48.0	53.6	38.3	759	165.0
Total for the day	147.5	75.7	85.8	1688	320.0

MENU G

BREAKFAST

	Carb	Prot.	Fat	Cal.	Mg.Na
4 oz. Orange Juice (½ c.)	11.3	.7		50	2.4
¼ c Oatmeal (1 oz.)	13.5	3.2	1.4	80	6.3
4 T. Cream (20%)	2.3	1.7	12.0	124	22.8
1 Slice Low Sodium Bread (Menu 1)	18.2	2.9	1.5	101	3.5
1 t. Butter			2.8	27	.2
Coffee with 1 T. Cream	2.3	.9	3.0	39	5.7
	47.6	9.4	20.7	421	40.9

LUNCH

	Carb	Prot.	Fat	Cal.	Mg.Na
Scrambled Egg and Mushroom (Menu 1) Substitute 1 T. Cream for Milk	.6	7.1	11.0	133	76.8
Salad. Crapefruit, 1 oz. Lettuce	5.5	.9	.1	28	4.7
Cherry and Banana Gelatin (Menu 21). Note: Use Standard can cherries in recipe. Do not use the Choice or Fancy Brands	25.8	2.0	.2	115	46.7
Coffee with 1 T. Cream	2.3	.9	3.0	39	5.7
	34.2	10.9	14.3	315	134.8

DINNER

	Carb	Prot.	Fat	Cal.	Mg.Na
½ lb. Boiled Liver	5.8	46.9	12.4	310	195.2
4 oz. Mashed Yellow Turnips	7.3	1.6	.2	40	5.6

	Carb	Prot.	Fat	Cal.	Mg.Na
Eggplant Mexican (Menu 21)	9.9	3.1	.7	57	23.2
Salad. 2 oz. Lettuce and 1 Medium Tomato	4.6	1.7	.7	31	10.0
Vinegar Dressing 4 t. 1 T. Vinegar and 1 t. Sugar	5.0			20	3.0
Pineapple and Coconut (Menu 3) Add	18.6	10.4	23.9	338	4.2
6 Soft-shell chopped Walnuts to this recipe	4.7	5.8	22.2	250	.6
Coffee with 1 T. Cream	2.3	.9	3.0	39	5.7
	58.2	70.4	63.1	1085	247.5
Total for the day	140.0	90.7	98.1	1821	423.2

MENU H

BREAKFAST

	Carb	Prot.	Fat	Cal.	Mg.Na
4 oz. Apricot Nectar	11.3	.6	.2	50	2.0
¼ c. Instant Ralston (1 oz.) with	21.0	4.5	.5	110	2
4 T. Cream	2.3	1.7	12.0	124	22.8
1 Slice Low Sodium Bread (Menu 1)	18.2	2.9	1.5	101	3.5
Coffee with 1 T. Cream	2.3	.9	3.0	39	5.7
	55.1	10.6	17.2	424	34.2

LUNCH

	Carb	Prot.	Fat	Cal.	Mg.Na
Spicy Creamed Egg (Menu 6)	8.0	10.1	14.0	215	106.5
1 Boiled Mashed Potato (3⅓ oz.)	18.0	2.2	.1	85	4.0
Salad, ½ Apple Sliced, ½ Grapefruit sliced on 1 Leaf Lettuce	11.6	1.1	.3	55	6.0
Coffee with 1 T. Cream	2.3	.9	3.0	39	5.7
	39.9	14.3	17.4	394	122.2

DINNER

	Carb	Prot.	Fat	Cal.	Mg.Na
Beef Stew (Menu 4) (2/3 to be eaten this meal, 1/3 may be used for Lunch)	28.8	48.4	36.2	652	227.1
Baked Potato, (5 oz.)	38.1	4.6	.1	175	10.0
1 t. Butter			2.8	27	2
2 oz. Hearts of Lettuce	.5	.6	.2	6	6.8
4 t. Vinegar Dressing (Menu 21)	5.0			20	3.0
Apple Sauce, unsweetened. Add	10.9	.3	.3	50	.4
Six Soft-shelled Walnuts, chopped	4.7	5.8	22.2	250	.6
Coffee with 1 T. Cream	2.3	.9	3.0	39	5.7
	90.3	54.8	42.6	969	253.2
Total for the day	185.3	79.7	77.2	1787	409.6

MENU I

BREAKFAST

	Carb	Prot.	Fat	Cal.	Mg.Na
4 oz. Grapefruit Juice (unsweetened)	10.2	.5	.1	45	.4
2 T. Farina (2/3 oz.) Do not use the quick cooking type	.0			l	
4 T. Cream (20%)	3	7	.0	4	.8
1 Slice Low Sodium Bread	.2	9	5	l1	5
1 t. Butter			8		
Coffee with 1 T. Cream	3		)	l	7
	48.0	8 2	19.5	406	32.7

LUNCH

	Carb	Prot.	Fat	Cal.	Mg.Na
1 Scrambled Egg in		6.7	5.2	75	67.0
1 t. Butter			2.8	27	2
2 oz. Spaghetti	45.1	7.2	2	219	4.4
Creole Sauce (Menu 7)	4.5	1.0	.4	26	5.0

	Carb	Prot.	Fat	Cal.	Mg.Na
Salad, 2 oz. Lettuce and ½ Sliced Orange with 3 chopped Walnuts	6.4	5.8	10.1	143	8.0
Coffee with 1 T. Cream	2.3	.9	3.0	39	5.7
	58.3	21.6	21.7	529	90.3

DINNER

	Carb	Prot.	Fat	Cal.	Mg.Na
Spanish Chicken (Menu 8)	25.7	57.4	18.6	506	193.3
French Fried Onions (Menu 8)	12.3	4.8	22.8	280	70.3
Boiled Potato (3⅓ oz.)	18.0	22	.1	85	4.0
Salad, 1 oz. Cabbage, 1 oz. Pineapple	4.2	.5		19	6.9
1 Slice Low Sodium Bread	18.2	2.9	1.5	101	3.5
Baked Apple (Menu 8)	12.2	.4	.5	55	2.6
1 T. Cream (20%)	.6	.4	3.0	31	22.8
Coffee with 1 T. Cream	2.3	.9	3.0	39	5.7
	93.5	69.5	49.5	1116	309.1
Total for the day	199.8	99.3	90.7	2051	432.1

SALT CONTENT OF 600 BASIC FOODS

INTRODUCTION TD TABLES

THE authorities referred to, were those available. A single glance across the table, quickly demonstrates the act that the definitive work in the field has yet to be done. The figures given by Henry C. Sherman and Peterson, Skinner and Strong, are usually far in excess of those quoted by the other two authorities. They are given, despite misgivings, as to their accuracy, because they have been so widely used and so long time-honored. McCance and Widdowson's figures are the result of careful chemical analysis, using the most recent chemical refinements. Mead Johnson's figures are obtained by the use of a flame photometer.

While there is occasional disparity between these last two authors, the magnitude of their differences is rarely as great as that between them and the other two authorities. We have used the higher figure in our computations as between McCance and Widdowson and Mead Johnson. Where no other figures are available, we have used those of Sherman or Peterson, Skinner, Strong.

It may be noted that with boiling, many foods lose some of their sodium. However, this loss is sustained only if the liquor in which the food was boiled, is not used. For example, an ounce of Spinach contains 54.2 mg. of sodium when fresh. After boiling, some sodium is dissolved in the liquor and the spinach contains only 34.9 mg. per ounce. To retain this loss, the liquor must not be used.

If there is disagreement between McCance and Widdowson and Mead Johnson on processed or canned foods, Mead Johnson's figures have been taken, since the foods tested by them are of American manufacture whereas McCance et al, have tested foods in England.

Following are tables giving the sodium and caloric values of food per ounce, and consisting of a comparative listing of the sodium content as given by:

(A)   R. A. McCance and E. M. Widdowson The Chemical Composition of Foods, 1947 Chemical Publishing Co., Inc., Brooklyn, N. Y.

(B)   Mead Johnson, Research Laboratory, 1947 Evansville 21, Ind.

(C)   Henry C. Sherman Ph.D., Sc.D. Chemistry of Food and Nutrition, 1946 The MacMillan Co., N. Y.

(D)   Peterson, Skinner, Strong Elements of Food Biochemistry, 1943 Prentice-Hall Inc., New York
In addition, the usual portions of food per person are given. Parenthesis signifies amount is variable.

Tr — trace.

Sodium is given in milligrams per ounce.

A ALE to BEANS

Food	Usial Portions	Cal	A	B	C	D
Ale, mild, bottled	½pt. – 8oz.	17	6.8	2.2		
Ale, pale, bottled	½pt. – 8oz.	19	48			
All-bran, Kellogg's	1 T. – 1/9oz.	88	(345)	400.0		
Allspice, ground				17.7		
Almonds	20 – 1 oz.	170	1.6	.5	7.4	6.8
Almonds, weighed with shells		63	.6			
Almonds, roasted in oil and salt				45.7		
Anchovy paste	1 t. – 1/5 oz.	60		3428.6		
Apple	1 -4¹/₃ oz.	10	.6	.02	2.8	4.2
Apple, dried	1 – 2 oz.	70				20.5
Apple juice	½ c. – 4 oz.	12		1.14		
Applesauce, canned	½ c. – 4½ oz	10		.09		
Apricots	1 – 5/6 oz.	8	Tr.	.14	8.5	6.0
Apricots, canned	½ c. – 4 oz.	17	.3	.5		
Apricots, dried	5 – 1²/₃ oz.	52	16.0			31.1
Artichokes,Globe or French	1 – 1²/₃ oz.				7.1	
Artichokes, Globe or French, boiled		4	4.2			
Artichokes, Jerusalem	1 – 3¹/₃ oz.	5	.7			
Asparagus	6 – 2½ oz.	5		.5	4.5	2.2
Asparagus, boiled			.5			
Asparagus, canned	6 – 2-5/6 oz	6		114.3		
Asparagus, frozen	6 - 2½ oz.	S'		.8		
Avocado	½ small – 2⁵/₆ oz.	25	4.6	.5	19.1	
Bacon	4 strips – 2²/₃ oz.	115	(348)	217.1	234.2	
Bacon, fried	4 strips –²/₃ oz.	142	(800)	914.2		
Bananas	1med. – 5oz	22	.3	.02	12.0	6.5
Bananas, weighed with skin		13	.2			
Barley, pearl	3 T. – 1 oz	102	.7	.85	16.0	
Barley, pearl, boiled	½ c. – 3¹/₃ oz.	34	.2			
Bass, steamed		36	21.3			
Bass, steamed, weighed with bone		19	11.3			
Beans, baked, canned	1 c. – 8 oz.	26	(168)			
Beans, broad, boiled	½ c. – 4¹/₆ oz	12	5.6			

Food	Usial Portions	Cal	A	B	C	D
Beans, butter	¾ c. -2½ oz.	76	17.4			
Beans, butter, boiled	½ c. -3⅓ oz	26	4.6			

B BEANS to BRAZIL NUTS

Food	Usial Portions	Cal	A	B	C	D
Beans, green	¼ - 3⅓ oz	50		.23		3.4
Beans, green, canned	½ c. - 3⅓oz.	6		117.1		
Beans, green, frozen	½ c. - 3⅓oz.	6		.5		
Beans, Haricot		73	*12.3*			
Beans, Haricot, boiled	½ c. - 4⅙ oz.	25	4.3			
Beans, lima, green	½ c. - 2½ oz.	38		.28		25.4
Beans lima, canned	½ c. - 4⅓ oz.	97		88.0		
Beans, lima, dried	½ c.. - 2½ oz..	106			47.7	80.5
Beans, Navy, dried	½ c.. - 2½ oz.	108		.26		
Beans, string	¾ c.. - 2½ oz.	4	1.8		6.5	3.4
Beans, string, boiled	2/3 c. - 4⅓ oz.	2	.9			
Beef corned, canned	¼ lb.	66	(392)	485.7		
Beef, dried	1/8 lb.	55		1114.2		
Beef, dripping	1 T. - 1/3 oz.	262	1.4			
Beef, frozen	½ lb.	43	21.0	15.1		
Beef, lean steak	½ lb.	50	19.6	15.0	24.0	18.8
Beer (see ale)						
Beets	2/3 c. - 3⅓ oz.	13		31.4	22.5	15.1
Beets, boiled	½ c. - 3⅓ oz.	13	18.2			
Beets, canned	½ c. - 3⅓ oz.	16		10.2		
Beets, leaves	1 c. - 3⅓ oz.	9		37.1		
Blackberries	½ c. – 2 oz.	8	1.1	.06	1.14	
Blackberries, stewed, no sugar	2/3c. – 4 oz.	4	.5			
Bloaters, grilled	¼ lb.	73	(200)			
Bloaters, grilled, weighed with bone		(54)	(148)			
Blueberries	2/3 c. - 3⅓ oz.	15		.14	4.5	
Bluefish	½ lb.	26			19.4	
Bouillon Cubes	1 – 1/7 oz.			7714.2		
Bovril	1 t. – 1/5 oz.	36	(1580)			

Food	Usual Portions	Cal	A	B	C	D
Brain, calf, boiled	¼ lb.	29	41.8			
Brain, pig	½ lb.	41		42.8		45.7
Brain, sheep, boiled	¼ lb.	31	48.3			
Brandy	1 oz.	75		.85		
Brazil nuts	4 - 1 oz.	183	.4	.23	7.4	
Brazil nuts, weighed with shells		82	.2			

B BRAZIL NUTS to CELERY

Food	Usial Portions	Cal	A	B	C	D
Brazil nuts, roasted in oil and salted				54.2		
Bread, Passover (see Matzoth)						
Bread, rye and wheat	1 sl. – 5/6 oz	72	(112)	160.0		
Bread, semi wholewheat	1 sl. – 1 œ	72	(112)	191.4		
Bread, white	1 sl. – 5/6 oz	75	(112)	191.4	127.4	147.7
Bread, wholewheat	1 sl. – 1 oz.	70	(112)	122.8		
Broccoli, tops	1 c. – 4 oz.	10		4.5	6.8	8.5
Broccoli, tops, boiled	½ c. - 3⅓ oz.	4	1.9			
Brussel sprouts	1 c. - 3⅓ oz.	16		3.1		
Brussel sprouts, boiled	½ c. - 3⅓ oz.	5	2.2			
Brussel sprouts, frozen	½ c. - 3⅓ oz.	5		2.5		
Butter, average salted	lxlx½ in. or	226		(280)		
Butter, lightly salted	1 T. melted - 1/3 oz.	226		(222.8)		
Butter, unsalted		226		1.4		
Buttermilk, cultured	1 c. – 8 oz.	20		37.1		
Cabbage, red	½ c. - 2⅚ oz.	6	9.0	1.4	9.1	10.8
Cabbagc, Savoy	1 c. – 4 oz	7	6.4	1.4	9.1	10.8
Cabbage, Savoy, boiled	½ c. - 3⅓ oz.	3	2.3			
Cantaloupe melon	3⅓ oz.	7	3.8	3.4	12.2	13.7
Cantaloupe melon, weighed with skin		4	2.4			
Caraway seed				4.5		
Carrots	½ c. - 2⅔ oz.	6	27.0	8.8	21.7	14.2

Carrots, boiled	½ c. - 2½ oz.	5	14.2			
Carrots, canned	2/3 c. -3⅓ oz.	12		80.0		
Cashew nuts	8 -½ oz.	171		3.7		
Cashew nuts, roasted and salted		200		57.1		
Catchup, tomato	1 T. – 2/3 oz	37		371.4		
Catfish	½ lb.	72		17.1		
Catfish, steamed	¼ lb.	34	30.6			
Catfish, steamed, weighed with bone		28	26.0			
Cauliflower buds	1¼ c. – 4 oz.	8		6.8	11.7	13.7
Cauliflower buds, boiled	2/3 c. - 3⅓ oz.	3	3.2			
Cauliflower buds, frozen	2/3 c. - 3⅓ oz.	3		6.2		
Caviar, Salmon	2 t. - ½ oz.	100		628.5		
Celery salt				7428.5		

C CELERY to CHICORY

Celery seed				40.0		
Celery stalks	2 stalks - 1⅓ oz.	3	38.9	31.4	37.1	28.8
Celery stalks, boiled	2/3 c. - 3⅓ oz.	1	18.9			
Cereal—all-bran	1 T. - 1/9 oz.	88	(345)	400.0		
Cereal, wheat. Instant Ralston	¼ c. - 1 oz.	110		.28		
Cereal, wheat. Maltex	¼ c. - 1 oz.	110		1.14		
Cereal, wheat. Pettijohn's	2 T. - 2/3 oz.	110		.5		
Cereal, wheat, Wheatena	¼ c. - 1 oz.	no		.28		
Chard, leaves and stalks	1 c. - 3⅓ oz.	8			24.5	
Cheese, American Swiss	1/8 in. sl. - 1 oz.	105		120.0		
Cheese, cheddar	1½x1½x1¼" - 5/6 oz.	120		154.2		
Cheese, cottage	¼ c. - 1⅚ oz.	36		91.4		
Cheese, cream	1/3 pkge. – 1 oz.	120		97.1		

Food	Usual Portions	Cal	A	B	C	D
Cheese, Dutch	1 oz.	77	(355)			
Cheese, Gorgonzola	1x½x2½" - ½ oz.	112	(347)			
Cheese, Gruyere	2x1x1" – 1 oz.	131	(154)			
Cheese, process				428.5		
Cheese, Parmesan	2 t. - 1/6 oz.	118	(215)			
Cheese, Stilton	1½x1½x1¼" - 5/6 oz.	135	(326)			
Cheese whey (cheese food)	1 c. - 7½ oz.	8		428.5		
Cherries, dark sweet	½ c. - 2½ oz.	13	.8	.28	.85	4.2
Cherries, dark sweet, weighed with stones		11	.7			
Cherries, dark sweet, canned	½ c. - 2-5/6 oz.	44		.2		
Cherries, dark, frozen in syrup	½ c. - 2-5/6 oz.	44		28		
Cherries, light sweet, canned	½ c. - 3⅓ oz.	aa 44		.85		
Cherries, glace	3- ⅓ oz.	60	18.4			
Chestnuts	8- 1⅓ oz.	49	3.1	.5	10.8	10.5
Chestnuts, weighed with shells		40	2.6			
Chicken, boiled	¼ lb.	58	27 8			
Chicken, boiled, weighed with bone		38	18.1			
Chicken, breast	½ lb.	46		22.2	26.0	15.4
Chicken₉ leg	½ lb.	47		31.4	26.0	15.4
Chicken, roast	¼ lb.	54	22.7			
Chicken, roast, weighed with bone	½ lb.	29	12.2			
Chicory	½ lb.	3	2.1			

C CHOCOLATE to CORN

Food	Usial Portions	Cal	A	B	C	D
Chocolate, milk	¾x1½x¼" – 1/5 oz.	167	(78)	24.5		
Chocolate, plain	¾x1½x¼" – 1/5 oz.	155	41)		16.0	5.4
Chocolate, syrup	2 T. - ½ oz.	80		.17		

Chocolate, unsweetened	½ oz.	180		1.14	
Cider, sweet applejuice	1 c. - 8 oz.	17		1.14	
Cinnamon, ground				2.2	
Citron, candied	¼ - 2½ oz	100		82.8	
Clams	6 – 2 oz.	25		51.4	172.4
Coca Cola	1 btl. - 6 oz.	10		.28	
Cocoa, ordinary	2 t – 1/6oz	128	(185)		
Cocoa, Hershey's				1.14	
Cocoa, powder, Dutch process	2 t. – 2 oz.			15.7	16.8	17.1
Coconut, dry	1½ c. - 3⅓ oz.	178	8.1	4.5	15.1
Coconut, fresh	1" sq. - 1/3 oz.	104	4.7		11.1	11.4
Coconut, milk	½ c. - 4 oz.	10	29.8		16.5
Cod	½ lb.	24		17.1	27.4
Cod, fillets, frozen	¼ lb.	24		114.3	
Cod, steamed	¼ lb.	23	28.4		
Cod. steamed, weighed with bones		19	23.0		
Cod liver oil	1 T. - ½ oz.	260		.02	
Cod roe, fried	2 oz.	59	36.0		
Cod, salted	¼ c. - 1⅔ oz.	54		2057.1	
Coffee	1 c. – 8 oz.	1	Tr.		
Corn, sweet white, canned	½ c. – 3-5/6 oz.	25		57.1	11.4
Corn, sweet white, milk stage	1 ear - 3⅓ oz.	33		.06	11.4
Corn, sweet yellow, canned	½ c. – 3-5/6 oz.	25		60.0	11.4
Corn, sweet yellow, frozen	1 ear - 3⅓ oz.	33		2.5	11.4
Corn, sweet yellow, milk stage	1 ear - 3⅓ oz.	S3		.09	11.4
Corn, yellow, dry				.11	
Cornflakes	1⅓ c. – 1 oz	104	(298)	188.5	
Cornflour	1 c. - 4⅓ oz.	100	14.7		10.2
Corn meal, yellow	1 T. - ½ oz.	110		.17	11.1
Corn oil	1T.-½ oz.	260		.06	
Com. popcorn, popped and oiled	1 c. - ½ oz.	120		.85	
Com. popcorn, popped, oiled and salted	1 c. - ½ oz.	120		428.5	

128

Food	Usial Portions	Cal	A	B	C	D
Cornstarch	½ c. - 2 oz.	110		1.14		
Cowpeas	2/3 c. - 3¹/₃ oz.	41		.28		
Cowpeas, dried	½ c. - 3¹/₃ oz.	105				10.2
Crab, boiled	2 oz.	36	104.0			
Crab, boiled, weighed with shell		7	20.7			
Crab, canned	½ c. - 3 oz.	23		285.7		
Cracker, graham	3 - 5/6 oz.	132		200.0		
Cracker, soda	3 - 1/3 oz.	135		428.5		
Cranberries	½ c. – 1²/₃ oz.	4	.5	.28	1.7	.5
Cranberry sauce, canned	1/3 c. – 3²/₃ oz.	55		.28		
Cream	1 T. - ½ oz.	115	9.0	11 4	(8.5)	8.8
Crisco	1 T. - ½ oz.	220		1.14		
Cucumber	2½x2" - 2½ oz.	3	3.7	.23	2.8	7.4
Currants, black	½ c. – 1²/₃ oz.	8	.8	.5	2.0	4.2
Currants, dried, black	1/3 c. – 1²/₃ oz.	69	5.5	6.2	5.1	21.4
Currants, red	½ c. – 1²/₃ oz.	6	.7	.5	2.0	4.2
Currantsf white	½ c. – 1²/₃ oz.	7	.4		2.0	4.2
Curry powder	1/5 t. – 1/60 oz.	67 18		12.8	48 0	
Dandelion	½ c. – 1²/₃ oz.	18		21.7		
Dates	3 - ½ oz.	70	1.4	.26	27.7	11.4
Dates, weighed with skin		61	1.2			
Dill, seed				3.4		
Duck, breast meat	½ lb.	48		19.4		
Duck, leg meat	½ lb.	48		27.4		

Food	Usual Portions	Cal	A	B	C	D
Duck, roasted	¼ lb.	89				
Duck, roasted, weighed with bone		48	29.8			
Eels, elvers	½ lb.	20	19.0			9.1
Eels, silver	½ lb.	90	21.8			
Eels, silver, weighed with bone and skin	½ lb.	60	14.5			
Eels, yellow	½ lb.	49	25.3			
Egg	1 av. - 1²/₃ oz.	46	38.4	40.0	40.0	31.7
Egg, white	1 av. – 1-1/6 oz.	11	54.7	57.1	48.5	50.0
Egg, yolk	1 av. - ½ oz.	99	14.2	9.7	16.0	22.2
Eggs, dried	1 oz.	165	147.0			
Eggplant	8 oz.	4	.7	.23	4.2	7.4

F ENDIVE to GRAPEFRUIT

Food	Usial Portions	Cal	A	B	C	D
Endive	¼ sm. hd. - ½ oz.	3	2.9	5.1	17.1	
Escarole	1/3 heart - 1²/₃ oz.	3			17.1	
Farina	2 T. - 2/3 oz.	105		.23	18.5	
Farina, quick cooking, enriched	2 T. - 2/3 oz.	103		28.5		
Figs, canned in syrup	3 – 3 oz.	50		.28		
Figs, dried	2 large - 1½ oz.	61	24.6	9.4	18.8	43.1
Figs, green	1 large - 1½ oz.	12	.5	.5	2.0	12.2
Filberts	20 - 1-1/6 oz.	214		.23		
Flounder	½ lb.	18			30.5	
Flounder, steamed	¼ lb.	27	32.6			
Flounder, steamed, weighed with skin and bones		15	18.2			
Flour, bleached enriched. Gold Medal	¾ C. - 3¹/₃ oz.	109		.28		
Flour, bleached, phosphated enriched	¾ c.- 3¹/₃ oz.	109		3.7		
Flour, buckwheat	1 c. – 4 oz.	102		.28	7.7	
Flour, gluten	¾ C. - 3¹/₃ oz.	103		.5		

130

Food	Portions	Cal	A	B	C	D
Flour, rye, dark	1 c. - $3^1/_3$ oz.	108		.28		
Flour, soya	1 c. - $3^1/_3$ oz.	84		.17		
Flour, white, natural	$3/4$ c. - $3^1/_3$ oz.	100	.6	.28	12.8	15.1
Force, whole wheat flakes	1 c. – 1 oz	115	(197)			
Frog's legs	½ lb.	19				15.7
Fruit salad, canned in syrup	1 c. - $4^1/_3$ oz.	20	.7	2.5		
Garlic	1 clove			1.7		2.5
Gelatin dessert, dry	¼ box - 5/6 OZ.	120		94.2		
Gelatin, plain	1 t. - 1/10 oz.	100		7.7		
Gin	1 oz.	75		2		
Ginger ale	1 c. - 7½ oz.	11		22		
Ginger, ground		74	10.0	8.2		
Gluten, wheat	$3/4$ c. - $3^1/_3$	103		.5		
Goose, roasted	¼ lb.	92	41.2			
Goose, roasted, weighed with bone		53	23.8			
Gooseberries	2/3 c. - $3^1/_3$ oz.	5	.5	.17	2.8	2.8
Grapes, black	20 - $3^1/_3$ oz.	17	.5		3.1	3.1
Grapes, white, seedless	30 - $3^1/_3$ OZ.	18	5	1.14	3.1	3.1
Grapejuice, sweetened, bottled	½ c. - 4 oz.			28		
Grapefruit	½ c. - $3^1/_3$ oz.	6	.4	.11	1.14	1.7

G GRAPEFRUIT to KIDNEY, BEEF

Food	Usial Portions	Cal	A	B	C	D
Grapefruit, whole fruit, weighed		3	.2			
Grapefruit juice, sweetened, canned	½ c. - 4 oz.	**17**		.11	1.4	
Grapefruit juice, unsweetened, canned	½ c.- 4 oz.	10		.11	1.4	
Grapenuts	¼ c.-1 oz.	102	(187)			
Gravy flavoring				24.5		
Haddock, fillets, raw	¼ lb.	20	35.5			28.2
Haddock, steamed		**28**	34.4			
Haddock, steamed,		21	26.2			

Food	Measure					
weighed with bone						
Haddock, steamed and smoked		**28**	346.0			
Halibut	½ lb.	**40**		16.0	31.7	
Halibut, steamed	¼ lb.	**37**	31.5			
Halibut, steamed, weighed with bone		**28**	23.8			
Ham, less excess fat	½ lb.	68		600.0		
Ham, boiled, lean	¼ lb.	**62**	(595)			
Hare, roasted	¼ lb.	**55**	15.0			
Hare, roasted, weighed with bone		**37**	10.2			
Hash, corned beef, canned	½ lb.	**34**		251.4		
Hazelnuts	20 - 1¹/₆ oz.	**214**			5.4	
Heart, beef	¼ lb.	**74**		25.7	43.7	29.1
Heart, sheep's, roasted	2 oz.	68	43.5	25.7	43.7	29.1
Heart, Turkey	1 oz.	**55**		19.7		
Herring	1 small - 3¹/₃ oz.	**67**	36.9			
Herring, roe, fried	2 oz.	**74**	24.6			
Hominy, canned	¼ c.- 1²/₃ oz.	**108**		51.4		
Honey	1 T. - 5/6 oz.	**82**	3.1	2.0	1.4	1.7
Honeycomb		**80**	2.0			
Horseradish	2 t. - 1/3 oz.	**17**	2.2			
Horseradish, prepared	1 T. - 1/10 oz.	*100*		27.4		26.8
Huckleberries	2/3 c. - 3¹/₃ oz.	**15**			4.5	
Ice Cream	1 gill - 2½ oz.	**58**	18.2			
Ice Cream, vanilla				28.5		
Jam. grape	1 t. - 1/3 oz.	**74**	4.5	2.0		
Jelly	1 t - 1/3 oz.	**73**	7.2			
Kale	1¾ c. - 6 oz.	**14**		31.4	14.8	14.2
Kidney, beef	5 oz.	**34**	69.5	60.0	65.7	68.0

Food	Usial Portions	Cal	A	B	C	D
Kidney, sheep	¼ lb.	34	71.0			
Kippers, baked	2 oz	57	281.0			
Kippers, baked, with bone and skin		31	152.0			
Kohlrabi	½ c. - 1²/₃ oz.	12			14.2	14.2
Lamb (see Mutton), less excess fat	1 ch. - 3¹/₃ oz.	53		31.4	24.0	14.0
Lard	I T. - ½ oz.	262	.6	.09		
Leeks	½ c. - 1-5/6 oz	7				10.2
Leeks, boiled	¾ c - 3¹/₃ oz.	7	1.8			
Lemons	1 - 3¹/₃ oz.	4	1.7	.17	3.7	2.5
Lemon juice	1 T. - ½ oz.	2	.4			
Lemon sole, steamed	¼ lb.	26	32.6			
Lemon sole, steamed, weighed with skin and bone		18	23.2			
Lentils	¼ C. - 2 oz.	84	10.2		16.2	
Lentils, boiled	½ c. - 3¹/₃ oz.	27	2.7			
Lettuce	2 lrg. lvs.-1²/₃ oz.	3	.9	3.4	8.5	8.0
Ling, steamed	¼ lb.	28	34.0			
Ling, steamed, weighed with bones		21	25.5			
Litchi, dried	8 lrg. pits - 5/6 oz.	90		.85		
Liver, beef		41	24.4		24.8	6.0
Liver, beef, fried	¼ lb.	81	26.1			
Liver, calf	½ lb.	57		31.4	24.8	
Liver, calf, fried	¼ lb.	74	34.6			
Liver, pig	½ lb.	39		22.0		
Liver, turkey	3¹/₃ oz.	42		14.5		
Lobster, boiled	1 av. - 3¹/₃ oz.	34	92.3	60.0		
Lobster, boiled, weighed with shell		12	33.2			
Loganberries	2/3 c. – 2½ oz.	5	.7		.5	
Loganberries, canned	2/3 c. - 4 oz.	29	.3			
Macaroni	½ c.- 2½ oz.			.28	5.1	28
Macaroni, boiled	1 c.- 2½ oz.	32	22			
Mace, ground				12.8		
Mackerel	½ lb.	41			43.7	
Mackerel, fried	¼ lb.	53	43.5			

| Mackerel, fried, weighed with bones | | 39 | 31.8 | | | |
| Malted milk | 1 T. - ¼ oz. | | | 125.7 | | |

Food	Usial Portions	Cal	A	B	C	D
Malted milk. Horlick's		114	196.0			
Maltex, see Cereals						
Maple syrup	1 T. – 3/5 oz.	85		4.0	3.1	
Margarine	1 T. - ½ oz	226	(90)	342.8		
Marmalade, orange	1 T . - 5/6 oz.	74	5.2	3.7		
Matzoth, American style	1-6" diam. - 2/3 oz.	105		102.8		
Matzoth, Egg				4.5		
Matzoth, farfel				8.0		
Matzoth, meal				1.14		
Matzoth, passover				.28		
Matzoth, plain				.28		
Matzoth, poppy seed				100.0		
Matzoth, wafer				122.8		
Matzoth, thin, tea				.5		
Matzoth, whole wheat				80.0		
Mayonnaise	1 T. - 2/3 oz.	225		171.4		
Melon, cantaloupe	¼-3¹/₃ oz	7	3.8	3.4	12.2	13.7
Melon, cantaloupe, weighed with skin		4	2.4			
Melon, yellow		6	5.5			
Melon, yellow, weighed with skin		4.0	5.5			
Milk, buttermilk, cultured	1 c. – 8 oz.	20		37.1		
Milk, evaporated	1 T. - ½ oz.	40		28.5		26.8
Milk, fresh, whole	1 c. - 8 oz.	19	14.2	14.5	14.5	13.4
Milk, whole dry	2 T. - ½ oz	150	113.0	117.1		99.4
Milk, goat	1 c. - 8 oz.	21		9.7		7.4
Milk, fresh, skimmed	1 c. - 8 oz.	10	14.8			
Milk, condensed,	1 T. – 5/6 oz.	100	40.7			

Food	Usual Portions	Cal	A	B	C	D
whole, sweetened						
Milk, condensed, whole, unsweetened	1 T. – 5/6 oz.	44	45.8			
Milk, human, from 4 mothers 49 to 77 days post-partum		20		3.1		
Milk, human, from 9 mothers 5 to 10 days post-partum		20		11.4		
Molasses, cane	1 T. - 5/6 oz.	80		22.8	12.2	
Mulberry	2/3 c. - 2½ oz.	10	.6	.17		
Mullet, steamed	2 av - 12/3 oz.	36	26.6			

Food	Usial Portions	Cal	A	B	C	D
Mullet, steamed, weighed with bone		23	17.0			
Mushrooms	½ c. - 1²/₃ oz.	2	2.6	1.4	7.7	3.7
Mushrooms, canne	½ c. - 2²/₃ oz.	Tr.		134.2		
Mussels	½ lb.	19	82.0			
Mussels, boiled		25	59.8			
Mussels, boiled, weighed with shells		7	17.9			
Mustard, prepared	1 t. – 1/3 oz	30		314.2		
Mustard, greens	½ c. - 1²/₃ oz.	3	5.4	13.7		5.7
Mustard, powder	1 t. – 1/6 oz.	132	1.0	.85		
Mutton (see Lamb)						
Mutton chop, grilled, lean	1 ch. - 3¹/₃ oz	77	36.0			
Mutton chop, grilled lean, weighed with fat and bone		36	17.0			
Mutton chop, grilled, lean and fat	1 ch. - 3¹/₃ oz	142	29.0			
Mutton chop, grilled, lean and fat, weighed with bone		108	21.8			
Mutton leg, boiled	¼ lb.	74	18.2			

Food	Usual Portions	Cal	A	B	C	D
Mutton, leg, roast	¼ lb.	83	20.1			
Mutton chop, raw, lean	½ lb.	53	25.9			
Mutton chop, raw, lean, weighed with bone		20	9.7			
Nectarines	1 - 4 oz.	14	2.6			
Nectarines, weighed with stones		13	2.4			
Nutmeg, ground				4.0		
Oatmeal	¼ c. - 1 oz.	115	9.5		20.2	20.5
Okra	7-2½" pods - 1²/₃ oz.	7		.28		
Oleomargarine	1 T. - ½ oz.	226	(90)	342.8		
Olives, green pickled	3 - ½ oz.	30	(639)	(628.5)	(339.7)	
Olive oil	1 T. - ½ oz.	264	Tr.	.06		
Olives, ripe, pickled	3 - ½ oz.	50		262.8		
Onions	1 med. - 2 oz.	7	2.9	.28	4.2	5.7
Onions, boiled	5 sm. - 2½ oz.	4	1.9			
Oranges	1 sm. - 3¹/₃ oz.	10	.8	.06	2.8	4.0
Oranges, weighed with peel and pips		8	.6			
Orange Crush, soft drink				.5		
Orange juice	½ c. - 4 oz.	11	.5	.11		1.7

O OVALTINE to PEPPER

Food	Usial Portions	Cal	A	B	C	D
Ovaltine	1 T. - 1/3 oz.	101	70.8			
Oyster	6 - .4 oz.	14	143.0	20.8	134.6	
Oyster, weighed with shells		2	17.2			
Pancreas, pig	3¹/₃ oz.	84		16.2		
Paprika, powder				23.4		
Parsley	1 t. - 1/30 oz.	6	9.4	8.0		
Parsnips, raw	¾ c. - 4 oz.	14	4.7	2.0	2.2	2.8
Parsnips, boiled	½ c. – 2²/₃ oz.	16	1.2			

Food	Usual Portions	Cal	A	B	C	D
Partridge, roast	½ c. – 2²/₃ oz.	60	28.4			
Partridge, roast, weighed with bone		36	17.0			
Peaches	2 - 5 oz.	11	.8	.02	4.2	3.4
Peaches, weighed with stones		9	.7			
Peaches, canned	2 halves - 4²/₃ oz.	19	.4	1.7		
Peaches, dried	3 - 1²/₃ oz.	61	1.7			20.0
Peaches, frozen	2 - 5 oz.			.85		
Peanuts	30 - 2 oz.	171	1.6		11.1	14.8
Peanut butter	1 T. - ½ oz.	190		34.2		
Peanut oil	½ c. - .4 oz.	267		.06		
Peanuts, roasted in oil and salted				131.4		
Peanuts, roasted in shell				.23		
Pears	1 - 4 oz.	12	.7	.5	2.2	2.8
Pears, weighed with skin and core		8	.5			
Pears, canned	2 halves - 4 oz.	18	.4	22		
Peas	½ c. - 2½ oz.	18	.1	26	5.4	6.8
Peas, boiled	½ - 2¹/₃ oz.	14	Tr.			
Peas, canned	½ - 2¹/₃ oz.	24	(74)	65.7		
Peas, dried	½ c. - 3¹/₃ oz.	78	10.8		25.4	
Peas, dried, boiled	½ c. - 3¹/₃ oz.	28	3.6			
Peas, frozen	2¹/₃ oz.			28.5		
Peas, split, dried	½ c. - 3¹/₃ oz.	86	10.9	12.0		
Peas, split, dried, boiled	½ c. - 4 oz.	33	4.0			
Pecan	6 whole - 1 oz.	185		.06		
Pepper, black ground (spice)		88	2.0	4.5		
Pepper, green (vegetable)	3" piece - 1 oz.	8		.14		4.2
Pepper, red (vegetable)						1.7

P PEPPER to POTATOES

Food	Usial Portions	Cal	A	B	C	D

Food	Portion					
Pepper, red. ground (spice)				13.1		
Pepper, white, ground (spice)				1.4		
Persimmon	1 small - 1²/₃ oz.	24		.23	3.1	3.7
Pettijohn's wheat cereal (see Cereal)						
Pheasant, roast	¼ lb.	61	29.6			
Pheasant, roast, weighed with bone		38	18.7			
Pickle, dill	1 med. - 1²/₃ oz.	3		657.1		
Pigeon, boiled	1 av. - 6 oz.	62	21.0			
Pigeon, boiled, weighed with bone		27	9.2			
Pigeon, roast	1 large – 2²/₃ oz.	66	29.8			
Pigeon, roast, weighed with bone		29	13.1			
Pike	½ lb.	24				8.2
Pineapple	1 c. - 5 oz.	13	.5	.09	4.0	2.2
Pineapple, canned	2 sl. – 5 oz.	18	.1	.28		
Pineapple, frozen				.28		
Pineapple, juice, canned, unsweetened	½ c. - 4 oz.	18		.11		
Plum	2 - 2 oz.	11	.5	.02	1.14	.85
Plum, canned	3 - 3¹/₃ oz.	35		5.1		
Pomegranate juice	½ c. - 4 oz.	13	.3	.09		
Popcorn, popped and oiled	1 c. - ½ oz.	120		.85		
Popcorn, popped, oiled and salted		120		428.5		
Pork, less excess fat	½ lb.	90	18.8	16.5	19.7	23.1
Pork chops, grilled, lean	1 chop - 3¹/₃ oz.	92	21.6			
Pork chops, grilled, lean, weighed with bone		38	8.8			
Pork chops, grilled, lean and fat	1 - 3¹/₃ oz.	155	16.8			
Pork chops, grilled, lean and fat, weighed with bone		128	13.9			
Pork leg, roast	¼ lb.	90	18.8			
Pork loin, roast, lean	¼ lb.	81	19.6			
Pork loin, roast, lean	¼ lb.	129	17.0			

and fat

Food	Portion	Cal	A	B
Pork loin, salt	2 oz.	240		828.5
Pork loin, salt and smoked	¼ lb.	69	511.0	
Postum, cereal beverage	1 t. - 1/15 oz.	105		10.2
Postum, instant, dry	1 t. - 1/15 oz.	90		20.2
Potatoes, chips	1⅓ c. - 1 oz.	175		97.1
Potatoes, sweet, boiled	1 med - 3⅓ oz.	23	5.1	

P POTATOES to RUTABAGAS

Food	Usial Portions	Cal	A	B	C	D
Potatoes, sweet, canned	2 small – 1½ oz.	90		13.7		
Potatoes, sweet, less skin	1-6" – 5 oz	36		1.14	7.7	8.8
Potatoes, white	1 med. – 4 oz.	24	2.0	.17	6.8	8.5
Potatoes, white, boiled		23	1.0			
Potatoes, white, canned				100.0		
Potatoes, white, fried		68	3.3			
Poultry seasoning				7.4		
Pretzels	6 med. – 1 oz.	95		314.2		
Prunes, canned	3 - 3⅓ oz.	30		.85		
Prunes, dried	8 lrg - 3⅓ oz.	46	3.5	1.4	22.2	28.8
Prunes, dried, weighed with stones		38	2.9			
Prune juice, unsweetened	½ c. –4 oz.	17		.5		
Pumpkin	¾ C. –4 oz.	4	.4	.11	15.4	3.1
Pumpkin, canned	½ c.–4 oz.	10		.5		
Quail. breast meat				100		
Quail, leg meat				12.5		
Quinces	1 – 8 oz.	7	.9	.17		
Rabbit, foreleg	½ lb.	35		13.4		13.4

Food	Usual Portions	Cal	A	B	C	D
Rabbit, loin	½ lb.	37		9.7		13.4
Rabbit, stewed	¼ lb.	51	9.1			
Rabbit, stewed, weighed with bone		26	4.6			
Radishes	6 med. – 1²/₃ oz.	4	16.8	2.3	18.2	23.7
Raisins	½ c. - 2½ oz.	70	14.9	6.2	24.8	34.2
Raspberry, black	2/3 c. - 2½ oz.	18		.06		
Raspberry, red	2/3 c. - 2½ oz.	7	.7	.11	.85	2.0
Raspberry juice	½ c. –4 oz.	14			1.4	
Rhubarb, raw	1 c.–3 oz.	2	.6	.28	4.8	2.8
Rhubarb, stewed without sugar	2/3 c. -3¹/₃ oz.	1	.4			
Rice flakes	1 c. – 1 oz.	120		205.7		
Rice puffed	1 c. - ½ oz.	120		.23		
Rice, polished and coated	1 T. - 2/3 oz.	102	1.8	.5	8.0	3.4
Rice, boiled	½ c. - 3²/₃ oz.	35	.6			
Rice, vitaminized		102		1.14		
Rum	1 oz.	75		.5		
Rutabagas	¾ c. - 3 oz.	14		1.4		14.8

R RYE to SPINACH

Food	Usial Portions	Cal	A	B	C	D
Rye flour (see Flour)						
Sage				5.4		
Sago	¼ c. – 1¹/₃ oz	101	1.0			
Salmon	8 oz.	60		13.7		
Salmon, canned	½ c. – 1¹/₃ oz	60	(152)	134.2		
Salmon, steamed	4 oz.	57	30.4			
Salmon, steamed weighed with hones		46	24.7			
Salt			11000.0	112₄₀.₅		
Sardines, herring, canned in oil	4-2½" long – 1²/₃ oz.	84	(223)	145.7		

140

Sardines, pilchard, canned in natural sauce	2 oz.	54	(169)	217.1		
Sardines, pilchard, canned in tomato sauce	3 oz.	40		114.3		
Sauerkraut, canned	2/3 c. - 3$\frac{1}{3}$ oz.	6		208.5		
Sausage, bologna	6 sl. – 2½ oz.	72		62.8		
Sausage, Frankfurt	2-7x¾" – 4 oz.	78		314.2		
Sausage, pork	2-3½" long - 1-1/6 oz.	97	(218)	314.2		
Sausage, pork, fried	2 oz.	93	(284)			
Scallops, steamed	½ c.- 3$\frac{1}{3}$ oz.	30	75.3			
Shortening, vegetable, Crisco	1 T. - ½ oz.	220		1.14		
Shortening, vegetable. Spry	1 T. - ½ oz.	220		.11		
Shredded Wheat	1 biscuit – 1 oz.	103	4.7	.5		
Shrimps	8 med – 3 oz.	32		40.0		
Skate, fried	4 oz.	69	51.8			
Skate, fried, weighed with bones		57	42.9			
Smelts, fried	3 - 3$\frac{1}{3}$ oz.	116	42.0			
Smelts, fried, weighed with bones		98	35.7			
Soda, baking, theoretical value for pure NaHCO3				7 320.8)		
Sole, lemon, steamed	4 oz.	26	32.6			
Sole, lemon, steamed, weighed with bones		18	23.2			
Soup, beef, canned, diluted as served	½ c. - 4 oz.	21		114.3		
Soup, tomato. canned, diluted as served	½ c. - 4$\frac{2}{3}$ oz.	18		114.3		
Soup, vegetable, canned, diluted as served	½ c. - 4$\frac{2}{3}$ oz.	24		42.8		
Soybean, dry	½ c. - 3$\frac{1}{3}$ oz.	120		1.14		
Spaghetti, see Macaroni						
Spinach	1¼ c. - 2½	6		54.2	24.0	26.5

oz.

Spinach, boiled   ½ c. - 3¹/₃ oz.   7   34.9

Food	Usial Portions	Cal	A	B	C	D
Spinach, canned	1 c. - 7½ oz.	7		85.7		
Spinach, frozen	1 c. - 7½ oz.	7		17.1		
Sprats, fried	2 oz	126	37.5			
Sprats, fried, weighed with heads		111	33.0			
Sprats, smoked, grilled	2 oz	91	(240)			
Sprats, smoked, grilled, weighed with heads		81	(213)			
Spry, see Shortening						
Squab, see Pigeon						
Squash, acorn	4 oz.	13		.09		3.1
Squash, hubbard	4 oz.	13		.06		3.1
Squash, yellow, summer	4 oz.	6		.14	.5	3.1
Squash, white	1¾ c. - 8¹/₃ oz.	6		.06		3.1
Strawberries	¾ c. - 3¹/₃ oz.	7	.4	.2	2.0	
Strawberries, frozen, sweetened	¾ c. - 3¹/₃ oz.	40		.5		
Sturgeon, steamed	4 oz.	44	30.6			
Sturgeon, steamed, weighed with bones		30	20.8			
Suet	1 T. - 1/3 oz.	262	6.0			
Sugar, light brown	1 T. - 1/3 oz.	105		6.8		
Sugar, while	1 T. - ½ oz.	112	.1	.09		
Sweetbreads, stewed	2 oz	51	19.6			
Sweet potatoes, sec Potatoes						
Syrup, chocolate	2 T. - ½ oz.	80		17.1		
Syrup, maple	1 T. - 3/5 oz.	85		4.0	S3.1	
Syrup, sorghum	1 T. - 2/3 oz.	75		5.7		
Syrup, tables, corn	½ c. - 5¹/₃ oz.	92		23.7		

and cane

Food	Portions	Cal	A	B	C	D
Tangerines	2-2" diam. - 3$\frac{1}{3}$ oz.	10	.6	.6		
Tangerines, weighed with skin		7	.4			
Tangerines, juice, sweetened, canned	½ c. - 4 oz.	12		.17		
Tapioca	¼ c. - 1$\frac{1}{3}$ oz.	102	1.2	1.4	1.14	
Tea (infusion)		Tr.	1.14			
Thyme, whole				10.2		
Tobacco, chewing				457.1		
Tomatoes	1 sm. - 4 oz.	4	.8	.85	5.7	3.7
Tomatoes, canned	½ c. - 4$\frac{1}{3}$ oz.	6		5.1		
Tomatoe juice, canned	½ c. - 4 oz.	6		65.7	42	
Tongues, beef	4 oz.	50		28.5		

R TONGUE to WHEAT

Food	Usial Portions	Cal	A	B	C	D
Tongues, beef, pickled	2 oz.	88	532.0			
Tongues, lamb, stewed	4 oz.	84	22.5			
Tripe, pickled	4 oz.	18		13.1		
Tripe, stewed	4 oz.	29	20.4			
Trout, steamed	4 oz.	38	25.0			
Trout, steamed, weighed with bones		25	16.5			
Trout, sea, steamed	4 oz.	37	58.7			
Trout, sea, steamed, weighed with bones		29	46.3			
Tuna, canned	½ c. - 3 oz.	87		154.2		
Turkey, breast meat	8 oz.	86		11.4	37.1	37.1
Turkey, leg meat	8 oz.	86		26.2	37.1	37.1
Turkey, roast	4 oz.	56	36.9			
Turkey, roast,		34	22.1			

weighed with bone

Food	Usual Portions	Cal	A	B	C	D
Turnips, white	¾ c. - 4 oz.	5	16.5	10.5	18.8	29.7
Turnips, boiled	½ c. - 4 oz.	3	8.0			
Turnips, leaves	1 c. - 3$^1/_3$ oz.	11		2.8	12.8	74.2
Turnips, leaves, boiled	½ c. - 3$^1/_3$ oz.	3	1.9			
Turnips, yellow, see Rutabagas						
Vanilla extract	1 t. - 1/6 oz.	12	.28			
Veal	8 oz.	31	30.4	13.7	25.4	24.5
Veal, frozen	8 oz.	31	27.0			
Veal, cutlet, fried	1 av. - 2$^2/_3$ oz.	61	30.1			
Veal, fillet, roast	4 oz.	66	27.5			
Venison, roast	4 oz.	56	24.4			20.0
Vinegar, cider	1 t. - 1/6 oz.	1	6.0	.28	5.7	
Vinegar, distilled				.17		
Walnuts, black	6 - 1-1/6 oz.	201		.5	6.5	3.7
Walnuts, English	6 - 1-1/6 oz.	156	.8	.5		
Walnuts, English, weighed with shells		100	.5			
Watercress	½ c. - 2/3 oz.	4	17.0		22.8	8.8
Watermelon	1 c. - 8 oz.	9		.09	5.7	3.4
Wheatena, see Cereal						
Wheat flakes	1 c. - 1 oz.	110		285.7		
Wheat germ, containing some bran and flour.				.5		
Wheat, puffed	1 c. - ½ oz.	110		.85		

W WHEAT to ZWIEBACK

Food	Usial Portions	Cal	A	B	C	D
Wheat, shredded	1 oz.	105	4.7	.5		
Whisky, blended	1 oz.	85		.09		
Whisky, bonded	1 oz.	85		.02		
Whiting steamed	1 oz.	26	36.1			
Whiting, steamed. weighed with bones		17	24.5			
Wine, port	1 wine gl. - 3$^1/_3$ oz.	49		1.14	2.2	
Wine, sauterne	3$^1/_3$ oz.	24		2.8		

Wineberry			.23
Worcestershire sauce	1 t. -1/6 oz.	24	400.0
Yeast, compressed	1½" sq – 3/5 oz.	25	1.14
Yeast debittered dry			51.4
Yeast, primary. cultured dry			8 to 520
Zwieback	1-3x1¼" - 1/6 oz.	120	71.4

CPSIA information can be obtained
at www.ICGtesting.com
Printed in the USA
BVHW041859140119
537812BV00012B/355/P